The Yoga
of Sailing

The Yoga of Sailing

DYANA WELLS

Anchors in an Open Sea trilogy
Book One

Fiery Scribes
PASSION-INSPIRED CREATIVITY

Author's disclaimer: Some names of people have been changed to protect identities. Nonetheless, the experiences of Alice and her family are based on true life.

Book and cover design by Brian Thurogood

Cover photograph by Raewyn Peart

ISBN 978-0-473-37386-3

Printed in New Zealand by Bookprinting.co.nz on recycled paper.

Copies can be ordered from retail booksellers or via

http://dyanawells.com

http://fieryscribes.com

DEDICATION AND ACKNOWLEDGEMENTS

Dedicated to my children: Laura, Sebastian and Madeleine.

ACKNOWLEDGEMENT FOR THE TRILOGY

Firstly, a big thank you to all my teachers, in particular Tarchin Hearn, Namgyal Rinpoche, Cecilie Kwiat and Lama Mark Webber. Without them, my life would have been very different and these books would never have been written.

I am very grateful to my mother, Margaret Peart, for her continued support for my writing over the last ten years and for her meticulous proofreading. She has helped me hold these stories right from the beginning to the end.

I am immensely grateful to Brian Thurogood, my dearest friend and editor, for his love and support and his endless constructive feedback which enabled these books to be completed and published.

Huge thanks to my father, Lindsay Peart, who took me away sailing and 'grew me up' on the land and ocean.

I am most appreciative of the patience and good spiritedness of my children, who joined me on many of the adventures in these stories. Sebastian, thank you for refining the voice of Oliver.

Thank you to all my students. You helped me hone my insights and provided a focus for the stories.

Many friends have read and helped me with my ideas and language, in particular Dido Dunlop, who had the first go at teaching me how to write, and Lisa O'Brien, who edited my stories in the early days.

Thank you to my creative writing teachers at Auckland University of Technology, in particular Mike Johnson and Stephanie Johnson. You made me believe my story could be told well.

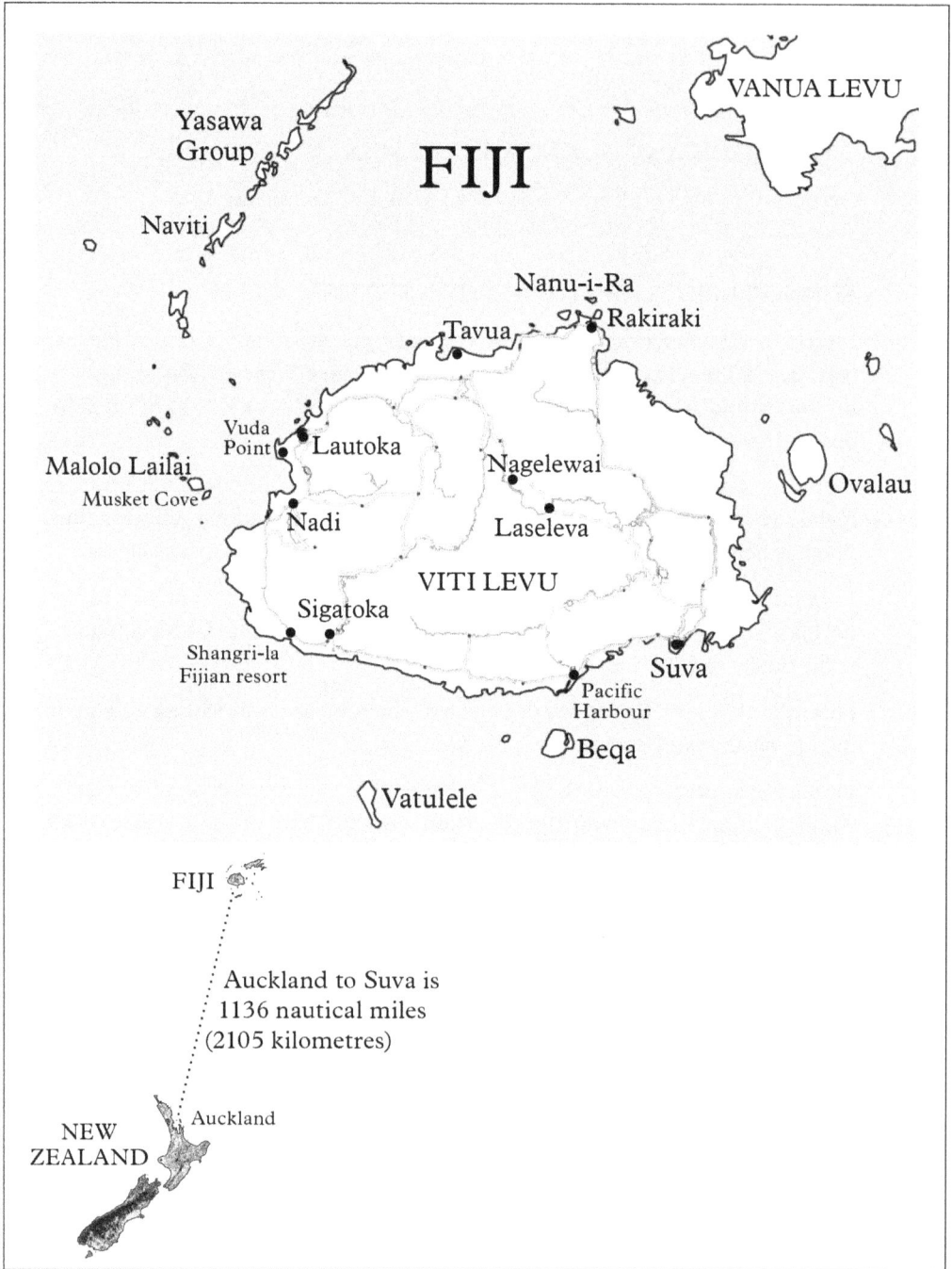

VANUA LEVU

Yasawa
Group

FIJI

Naviti

Nanu-i-Ra

Tavua

Rakiraki

Vuda
Point

Lautoka

Nagelewai

Malolo Lailai

Ovalau

Musket Cove

Nadi

Laseleva

VITI LEVU

Sigatoka

Suva

Shangri-la
Fijian resort

Pacific
Harbour

Beqa

Vatulele

FIJI

Auckland to Suva is
1136 nautical miles
(2105 kilometres)

Auckland

NEW
ZEALAND

PART ONE

1

'Mum, can you bring me a glass of juice?' Emily pleads from her berth. This time I'm lucky – I get to the galley unbruised. Still standing, I wedge myself in tightly so my hands are free to work the pump. 'Won't be long. Jack, would you like one too?' I ignore the nausea washing through me with every roll and wait for a still moment between rolls and the crash of the boat falling off another wave. I fill the glass. Now I have to get it to her before it ends up in a mess on the floor.

We're pushing into a forty-five knot storm-force wind. The wind's been thirty-five knots for the last three days. That's gale force. We're heading for Tonga, an archipelago of Pacific islands north-north-east of us. We keep *Dream-maker* pointing as close to the wind as she can. A large anticyclone is moving north-east with us, at the same speed. We're in the back of it, around the ten o'clock point. Just our luck! If we'd been on the other side we'd be speeding to Tonga, down-wind all the way.

Dad, Emily's seventy-seven-year-old grandad, is on watch in the cockpit, waterproofed from head to foot, safety-harnessed to a stainless cleat. *Dream-maker* is a dry boat – she doesn't take much water over the deck, yet huge cold waves break over the bow and wash across the deck and cabin top. Most of them miss him. Around the open rear cockpit the sea churns and foams dangerously close all the time.

I'll be sailing offshore for the first time. I'm forty-seven years old and my three children have grown up enough for me to make a fresh start. I've been riddled by deeper questions for many years. Being alone on watch in the middle of a vast ocean seems a good place to fish for answers. I'm watching Dad carefully. There's a lot of him in me. Dreams of romance and adventure fill both our ragged sails. We're both restless; I need to find out why. I'm expecting great things from this trip. I need some answers because my life doesn't work too well.

Like all modern sailing boats, *Dream-maker* accomplishes the miracle of sailing into the wind. Her sails belly out, creating a vacuum on the leeward side as wind rushes past. The vacuum sucks the boat forward the same way it lifts an airplane into the sky. I find it hard to believe the vacuum theory, but it's all I have. I'm always on the lookout for good theories, physical and metaphysical.

The wind shrieks and howls, not letting up for an instant. Tight sails strain against the fury, shuddering, not daring to let go. I wonder something doesn't break. I'd be scared if I let go trust in Dad for a second. We've been in a wintry sea for a week, with huge wind-tossed seas bearing down on us. *Dream-maker* doesn't seem to mind. Like a toy in a lumpy bathtub of childish delight, she climbs up one wave and crashes down over its crest; then she ploughs part way through the next, only to be blown aside by the wind. On and on, she bashes and crashes. Dad has total confidence in her ability to get us there. I fear her fibreglass hull may shatter. Her liveliness makes it almost impossible for me to do anything inside the boat. I steady myself in the galley before setting off for the saloon. Feet solidly planted, I sway and curve like a doll of wooden beads and elastic. I take a tentative first step.

I wanted this adventure. Ten days ago, Dream-maker was tied up in a marina in New Zealand and I was alone in the cockpit, watching the sky shadow through purples and golds. The reflection in the sea broke masts and stays of nearby yachts into bits and pieces and I followed the tinsel of shore lights through the water. We were getting ready to leave. Everything we needed had been dumped in the saloon for me to stow, but the cupboards were already full. I stared glumly at barely-holding-together bags and boxes of food, duty-free alcohol, roughly-folded duvets and sheets, a deflated plastic dinghy crumpled in a corner, rusty tools and smelly containers of diesel. The last threads of sunlight winked off the golden teak.

Months ago now, we re-glassed the hull. Dad was master of ceremonies as we held sheets of soft, prickly fibreglass against the hull and rolled on thick acrylic resin. An enthusiastic gathering of children, grandchildren and sailing friends, we splashed globs of resin onto the oil-stained ground and paint tins and brushes that lay around. We covered ourselves and the boat in threads of sticky glass, then stopped for fluffy cheese-bread and tea.

The place was full of old caravans and boats, a depressing scrap yard of abandoned dreams. Rust and dry rot had swallowed the hopes and money of many a rum-soaked captain. Dad was determined to leave. After weeks of sanding the lumpy fibreglass, he sprayed it a proud royal blue. He and I rolled on the antifouling, following the masking tape for a neat line. He had a new list every week. I trotted a broken stanchion to the garage for welding. I learned to re-solder and shrink-wrap electrical connections that had oxidised and broken in the salt air. We sanded, painted, screwed, cleaned and untangled wire stays that would hold up the mast. I fixed the navigation lights. The mast was not yet on the boat and I wondered how it would get there.

Finally, *Dream-maker* was ready for launching. We needed a spring tide to float her clear of the mud. One day, a trolley arrived and trundled her down to the water. She left three uncertain years behind in a halo of empty paint tins. Dad motored across the harbour to a marina berth in West Auckland. After the mast was stepped he fixed the stays and bent on the sails. She was back in the sea, ready to go.

She's a standard 36-foot Westerly ketch with a second aft mast. Two dark narrow quarter-berths in the stern hug both sides of the cockpit, smelly old diesel engine in between. The berth behind the galley on the starboard side is mine, and the one on the port side behind the navigation table is Dad's. In the galley is a two-burner gas stove, a defunct gas oven, a sink with a fresh water pump and a rusted-up salt water pump. The boat is old but seaworthy again – just. Charts, navigation instruments, the GPS and peeling radio boxes sit snugly above the navigation table opposite the galley. I walk through the saloon with its fixed mahogany table and comfortable settee-like bunks on either side, where Emily and Jack will sleep. Food, tools, books and clothes are stuffed under, behind and above the settees. Opposite the head (toilet) at the for'ard end of the saloon is a large wardrobe, filled mainly with my gear. The fo'c'sle, at the front of the boat, has a cosy double bunk with the chain locker in front – Dad's bed until yesterday – not a good place to sleep in the open sea because of the movement.

We're almost ready to leave. Emily, my 23-year-old daughter, fine hair sprouting from a clean head shave a month ago, and Jack, her slimline red-haired boyfriend, arrive trundling their gear along the pontoon. I don't know where to put it. The cupboards and fo'c'sle bunk are already full up with my bicycle, its panniers, two tents, a fish smoker, crab net, pack, sleeping bag, cooker and a second rubber dinghy. Dad has dumped his new computer (a bulky PC), LCD screen and scanner (for transferring old slides to CD) on the bunks in the saloon. Emily and Jack drop all their gear in the cockpit for now. We have two days altogether – tied up to the marina berth – for the last-minute scramble.

Emily remembers all the reasons for not going. 'This is a dangerous crossing.' 'Grandad and his boat are old.' The muddle doesn't inspire her. 'What about seasickness and sleepless nights? Can I still change my mind?'

I send her back into the city for last-minute purchases.

'We can get away tomorrow,' I reassure Dad.

'Emily, take the gas bottles to the garage and fill them. Jack, here's the prescription for our drugs.' Don't know what he's thinking; he doesn't say much. 'Emily, you and Jack will need your own snorkelling gear, so get that now. I'm going to the bank to get a visa card.'

'Mum, you're too late. It takes days.'

'We need Polaroid glasses for coral spotting. Let's go together.'

It's almost over.

'Alice, I don't think we can do it, we need more time,' Dad pleads.

He hands me another list. In my experience, the muddle dissolves once the adventure begins. I don't give an inch.

'It's okay, you'll see. We can do it. What else do you want done?'

We make a final list. We can do it.

Dad will be sailing offshore for the seventh time. Each time he staggers home exhausted, like the ancient mariner – heavily-creased forehead, hair stiff with salt, face bristling white surrender – declaring his retirement from sailing. He soon forgets the hardship and loneliness, though. Now he's springing around the boat like someone half his age.

We had a family farewell last night, at my sister Marion's new home, an old villa in Ponsonby. She'd just had it opened up inside, re-gibbed and freshly painted. My mother emerged from a deep leopard-skin-patterned sofa on the other side of the room and set off for the kitchen to refill her glass with half wine, half grape juice. Sipping the impotent mix, she glanced up at a disturbing painting of slaves and slave traders that Marion had brought back with her from South Africa, then crossed the oriental-style rug to join us. She's lived on her own now for fifteen years, in a neat townhouse with a small garden and small view of a lagoon that has many water birds. At home this evening, she plucked her eyebrows to a gracious curve and filed her nails to a neat team of waning moons. She smiled at me and Marion and didn't say a word. She's spent more than twenty years reading new age books and her fridge is covered in affirmations to remind her how wonderful life is. She can have anything she wants as long as she believes she's worth it.

Marion offered Mum the cashews, then slipped into the kitchen to take out the pizzas. She returned, still holding a tea towel.

'Congratulations. Well done,' she smiled and bashed my shoulder affectionately. 'I'm surprised you made it this far. I thought Dad was done for, holed up in Spam Farm with his old cronies, channel silting up and mangroves creeping up the slipway. I'd say you dragged him away just in time. You'll have trouble getting him away from Tonga once you arrive though,' she continued confidently. 'When I sailed with him ten years ago he definitely wanted to stay put.'

Gunshot exploded from the kitchen and a bottle of bubbly frothed into outstretched glasses.

'I wonder why you never explored spirituality,' I asked Marion, ignoring the outrageous possibility of 'staying put' anywhere. 'You're the only one in the family not to.'

Mum looked up, forming my question on her face, her wan smile hovering between a grimace and sympathetic interest.

'Hmmmm ... ' Marion started hesitantly. 'The outside world fascinates me.'

Mum bravely held her smile while she did a disappearing act inside her purple cardigan and matching purple pants. Someone over in the corner changed the music and Neil Young lifted us into a melancholic redemption.

Dad arrived, polo shirt tucked into loosely-belted jeans, canvas boat shoes padding over the rugs, glowing with family pride.

'I'm doing pretty well to be sailing at my age,' he started out. 'Life is a wonderful adventure. I'm bringing some tapes of Ramtha, Alice, you might like to listen to them on the way over.'

He turned to Marion, who's been out of his loop of inspired discourses by Ramtha.

'Ramtha is a channelled entity who reminds us that we are gods like him. We can have any life we want – the power and freedom are with us.'

He didn't flinch saying this or squirm thinking more of an explanation might be needed.

'Dad, you don't seem to have a dilemma fitting ordinary life and spirituality together?'

'Not at all. Spiritual teachings opened out my life in a way I could never have imagined. The spiritual and the ordinary aren't separate.' He slowed. 'Spiritual laws are natural laws. When you understand them they give you control over your life, they give you more choices, that's all.'

Mum looked at Dad, fingering the buttons on her cardigan, looking around as if about to flee, repeating her inner mantra, "Thank heavens I'm not still married to him."

'Well,' Dad continued, after grabbing a handful of nuts, 'You Buddhists get all hung up on suffering. Life isn't about suffering.'

Emily, my eldest daughter, wandered over, cautiously curious. She grew up when I was always rushing off to another spiritual retreat or evening or weekend. Her father accused me of being selfish and self indulgent. He claimed my spiritual interests obsessively missed the point. My problems were emotional not spiritual, he'd said, and my retreats were a way of not facing them or him. Emily didn't know what to think. Maybe her dad and I would still be together if I hadn't gone off like I did.

My arm crept around her waist. She's been my steady companion since the end of my marriage. Now she wants to break free and find out who she is without me. She wasn't at all sure about the sailing trip, but at least she can fly home with Jack if she's miserable. She listened to the conversation, soaking it up with one ear and rejecting it angrily with the other. Jack, her boyfriend, sat near the door all evening, pretty much on his own, drinking beer. Charlotte, my youngest daughter, kept him company recounting stories about drunken friends. I returned to the kitchen for more wine.

The morning of our departure arrives. One wave at a time, Tonga is 1000 nautical miles away. We have from May until November to cruise the South Pacific. The cyclone season, when most of the boat-capsizing, mast-breaking storms blow, starts in November. We motor out of the marina into the Waitemata Harbour. Emily, Jack and I are a tentative crew. We cross the Hauraki Gulf – daytime recreational waters for Auckland sailors – and head for the tip of the Coromandel Peninsula. The boat sails well, which is good. Several hours pass.

Dad points out Tryphena harbour on a chart of Great Barrier Island.

'We'll go in here for the night, so we can get the boat shipshape and find our sea legs.' He hands Jack a beer and sits down with him.

'Well, Jack, this is your last chance to leave. We're heading straight for Tonga tomorrow. The ferry back to Auckland goes in the morning.'

Dad is joking, almost. Jack doesn't look too good.

He cringes slightly and turns away to hide his thoughts. "Was agreeing to this trip a big mistake? Would I be chickening out if I left now?" He is only just a man at twenty-four and doesn't know anything about sailing.

I dive into our new situation with exaggerated confidence. I cook and re-stow our stores. Dad radiates an air of global acceptance. He's the only one with any clue about what lies ahead. Emily's mood I hardly notice; I take her willingness to be here for granted.

On the evening of our second day at sea, the last shadows of land fade. We're alone in the great ocean. The moody ocean is no place for Jack. Emily's resigned – to what she's not quite sure. Dad's busy with the radio, fiddling the knobs. He checks the wires and connections again; all he gets is crackling and a pale green light. Auckland Cruising, a team of volunteers on shore who follow cruisers and forecast the weather, expect us to call in with our position and course. They're our safety net.

The sea turns to glass, cheerily reflecting the stars, as we roll helplessly in the swell, rigging jangling, sails hanging loose. Not moving at all is about as bad as it gets for me. Fortunately, a new wind comes up and we're off again.

'Mum, I can't eat. I don't feel well, neither does Jack.'

Emily hands back half-eaten meals. They slouch on watch, then crumple up on their bunks. They don't talk, even to each other. Dad doesn't look happy either. Maybe he's frustrated with the radio and the lack of general order?

'They'll get over their seasickness. Emily is normally very helpful,' I reassure him.

'Seasickness can be a serious problem,' he warns. 'I heard of one woman who was airlifted off a yacht because she was so sick.'

I'm happy to be here, doing something exciting. I left work six months ago, burnt out, all brain fuses blown, and after months of recuperating, I turned into a roving handyman, never sleeping more than a few days in the same place. I worked on Dad's boat, helped Mum paint her kitchen and bathroom, did renovations on my seaside home at Orere Point and fibreglassed the deck of a rental property I have in town. A roving handyman is not the sort of person I want to be. *Dream-maker* is a haven of stability. I need to find my way back to deep stirrings that meant everything to me many years ago.

Four days of sailing and my head starts hammering loudly. I creep into my quarter berth to die, but I can't leave Dad alone. Emily and Jack are seasick around the clock. I can't be sick, and that's all there is to it. I climb down gingerly in the morning and swallow two Panadol – they have no effect. Dad hunts down a triple-strength prescription pain-killer – it works.

Dad is rock-solid, good-humoured and methodical. He knows the ocean. I follow him up on deck and pull at pieces of rope with strange names like halyard and sheet. He doesn't sleep or eat much; none of us eats much. He studies the clouds and sea, frowns and resets the sails.

After six days, we've covered 400 nautical miles with 600 to go. That's slow, an average speed of 5-6 knots, about 10 kilometres an hour. Twice a day, with dividers and pencil, I plot co-ordinates from the GPS onto the chart, with small crosses close together making a jagged trail across the Pacific. The wind's still blowing across the bow, almost directly from Tonga. We can't hold the most direct course. If we turn any further into the wind, the sails will collapse. I don't want to tell Emily and Jack how slow progress is.

'Mum, what will I do when I run out of sea sickness pills?' She rushes out to vomit over the side. 'Jack's headache is worse. He's going to die. How far have we got to go?'

I go over to Jack. 'Here's a sleeping pill – take it. You need a break – I'll do your watch.'

He stares back, greenish-white behind the freckles and limp movements, and shakes his head. Ashen and gaunt, he drags himself into the cockpit and slumps under the dodger to wait out his three-hour watch, every now and then hanging over the side to throw up, too despairing to put on his harness. A boarding wave could send him over as well. A wispy ghost-like voice rises up from below offering him crackers.

Day follows day in the same unhappy way. Eventually Jack confesses in a raspy voice: 'I'm in the recurring nightmare of my childhood. In my dream I'm on a small boat in the middle of the sea. The boat is about to sink with me in it.' He tries to smile. 'There's nothing I can do. My nightmare is going to come true. I know. I shouldn't have come.'

He collapses back down to his bed.

Holding the glass of juice for Emily, I grab the end of the navigation table to steady myself. The boat plunges down, the juice lifts off from the glass and sprays over the already coffee-stained chart. My stomach lurches; I swallow hard and grab a cloth from the sink. My legs flex and wobble. I could give up, but I can't. I lurch back into the galley, wedge myself in tightly and pour another glass. Emily and Jack would probably recover if we had a break from the movement and noise. Water sloshes around in the toilet bowl like someone's throwing up all the time.

Going to the toilet is almost impossible in a rough sea. Emily opens the heavy teak door. It pulls free and swings wildly open and shut, banging. Gripping her knees around the toilet, elbows wedged against the walls, she pulls her trousers down. Her stomach heaves but she resists the impulse to turn and put her face down the bowl. Finally she wipes her bottom without losing her balance, crashes into the basin, and drags her trousers up with one hand. Forget about washing hands.

I jump with relief when Dad calls, 'Alice, we have to put up the storm sail.' I pull on my raincoat and waterproof pants. 'I don't think the main will hold up in this wind,' Dad yells, almost drowned out by the wind. 'Put on your harness.'

First I clip on my new self-inflating lifejacket, which I bought especially, and attach the ragged safety-halyard, first to the lifejacket and then to the boat. Dad uses a thirty-year-old piece of tied rope for his halyard. Fighting against the wind and spray, we drag the storm sail on deck and tie it to the boom. I release the main and try to tug it down. Then I grab clumps, nails breaking, and pull with all my weight. The wind forces the sail against lazy jacks, which are meant to make dropping a sail easy. We shackle the small orange tri-sail to the halyard. I winch it up until Dad shouts 'Stop,' and then cleat it tightly against the mast. This physical work of sailing is exhilarating.

I soak up the good outside sounds, like the howling wind, rising and falling, adding a piercing whistle when it finds a hole to blow through. It's roaring now, racing the boat through the waves. The headsail adds to the symphony with a rebellious flap – it often does this because it's old and doesn't set well. The sea crashes and sometimes gently laps, adding a constant tenor to the chorus. Rigging rattles and chimes all the time. The different voices come together and then stray apart, crying their song to no one in particular.

After a week at sea, my rubber sea legs wobble steadily through the rolls and crashes. I decide to wash the dishes – there aren't many, even after a week. I pump a little water in the bottom of the sink. Any more than a couple of inches will fly out in the next boat roll.

It's time to fix the stove which is hanging uselessly in the corner – it came off its brackets days ago. Wedged into the corners of the galley, I hold it up while Dad gets in behind.

'Looks like a screw's come out,' he calls. 'Easily fixed. Can you hold it for a bit longer?'

'Sure.'

The kettle is soon boiling and I spoon powdered mushroom soup into everyone's thermos cups.

Dad returns to the radio. The transmitting signal is still very weak. His boat is a junk yard of old, second-hand equipment that needs constant coaxing and tweaking. He knows what to do, though. He's from the generation that can fix anything: plumbing, mechanical, electrical or metaphysical. He's been on the inside of all his equipment many times.

Jack's on his bed, waiting for the end, and discards his soup after a few sips. Tightening a loose screw won't be enough to fix him.

'Mum, I've used up all grandad's pills now. What will I do?'

'I don't know.'

She glances over to Jack. He can't save her. They've only been together a month or two. How did she end up here with her mum and grandad on this beastly boat?

'I'm cooking scrambled eggs with bacon for lunch.'

With Emily's encouragement, Jack eats a little. Dad eats alone in the cockpit, staring into space.

When I was young, Dad rebuilt two trimarans from dry, rotted shells. Every summer our family sailed up and down the coast of New Zealand. I never learned to sail – I just did what I was told. Now Dad explains everything we do, slowly and clearly, until I understand. I take over radioing our position and speed to Auckland Cruising every night.

Dad looks up from studying the chart and the GPS. 'Alice, I know you're not going to want to hear this, but we can't get to Tonga. The wind's directly on the nose. It's too hard on Jack and Emily and on the boat. We'll head for Fiji.' Emily and Jack look relieved. 'However, it will take us a few more days to get there.'

The groan from Jack is long and desperate. 'I can't last that long. This is too terrible.'

Emily would panic if it would help. On our new course, heading as far into the wind as we can, we'll only just make Fiji, far to the west of Tonga.

Outside, the weather is changing. The wind has settled down to twenty-five knots with a three-metre swell. We've crept up to a latitude of 25 degrees, so it's warm and the sky is a gentle misty-blue. During long solitary hours on watch, I gaze into the hazy horizon where the sky and sea dissolve together. I gaze into the sky, streaked with greyish-brown, like wild geese making their way home somewhere. I melt into beauty.

My relationship to life is changing. I had forgotten this great mysterious creature, 'life'. She is calling me. She whispers, reminding me why I came away with my father on this boat – I came to meet her. When I turn over the question, 'What is the meaning of my life?', she appears in my heart as a wild, gentle presence and grows outside of me, huge and beautiful. When I am alone in vast nature, slipped away from my thoughts and plans, I recognise a different kind of relationship, one that connects me to her.

I remember pencil crosses marking my journey, the way I sailed in search of her. At school, I was in love with numbers and the beauty of scientific explanations. When I solved chemical and mathematical equations, organic, planetary resonances shivered inside me. I peered into the spiral-hearts of flowers, wondering if the curves travelled inwards forever. I slipped along xylem and phloem in the quietly reverent way plants seem to do. I devoured as many textbooks as my father could bring home from teacher's training college, where he was a lecturer. At university, I majored in botany and zoology. I was looking for answers to the 'what is the meaning of my life?' question. I found none, because she was separate from me, on the outside. Though the scientific descriptions of her forms were rich and detailed, I wasn't in the picture; I wasn't part of her beauty.

I started a second and third degree in philosophy. Thought became the next pencil cross in my search for meaning. I studied treatises of German idealism, modern existentialism, philosophies of religion and theories of knowledge. I was trailing a small tribe of children by now. I lay in the bath, infant asleep on my breast, heavy philosophies of Kant and Schopenhauer propped on my island knees. Maybe these books would show me a place to live that wasn't in my head. The ivory tower of philosophical analysis turned into a tortured game of thesis and antithesis.

I shook water droplets from the book covers and wrapped my babe in a towel. Western academia was a dead man's land. I did glimpse 'her' in some of the pages. I could tell the great philosophers were men of knowledge. They had explored far more than the logical structure of an argument. Their ideas had grown from places deeper than my teachers had ventured, but I couldn't get there by myself.

I unrolled my chart again to find not so many routes left. I plotted my next cross: spirituality. I didn't even know what the word meant. I had always resisted gullibility, superstition and esoteric glamour. This cross scared me. I had explored the far reaches of Western thought and found them barren – l had no choice but to head east.

My family watched me slip away. The rational cliff edge I had been standing on my whole life crumbled and I fell far away from everything I had known, into the arms of mystery. I focused my well-trained mind on the subject of experience, the 'I.' My feet touched solid rock. I gained a glimpse of who I was, for the first time in my life. I met truth, the promised land. There was nothing to do but put out more sail. I was sure of success, I was sure I could stay in the arms of mystery and never return. I would make this mystery my home. My heart burst with such longing I thought I would break apart.

Wind rips past the sails. I gaze into the beauty of the indigo sky. 'What is the meaning of my life?' I ask the question again for the first time in many years. The question breaks up in the spray, while I squirm and refold myself in a different way. I'm making a fundamental error. Salty droplets of insight land on my face. I'm starting at the beginning again, hunting life's meaning in the wrong place, in the thinking place. This question grew from a place behind my thinking mind, and ended up in a thought. On this trip, I want to explore the subtle byways of my feelings, I want to be still and open enough to find my way into a quality of knowing that doesn't hold onto words. I want to find my way back to her, this beautiful mysterious creature I call *life*. This is where my quest to bring the ordinary and mystical together will begin. I have plenty of time.

2

Jack's face is twisted in agony, living his nightmare – shipwrecked at the bottom of the sea – waiting for it to happen, an inner mantra of torture running on and on: 'Why didn't I get off at Great Barrier? I knew I shouldn't have come.' Every minute is intolerable.

Dad disappears behind a bristling white beard and hovers around the outskirts, either in the cockpit or his bunk. We are all locked up inside ourselves. When he comes out to take over my watch, I go down to make him tea with crackers and cheese.

'Thanks, Alice.'

His soft blue eyes are almost transparent, his gentle face washed clear by the sea. I hardly know my father and now he's old. We sit in the cockpit across from each other. He's cross-legged, one foot swinging slightly and the other solidly planted. His long sculptured toes have always fascinated me, with their gnarly claw-like nails which he has to saw because they're too tough for scissors or clippers. His arms fold tightly across his chest. Behind the frustrations though, he's all given up to the sea. He can get us to Fiji easily.

He's lived part-time on *Dream-maker* for the last ten years, tending to her: patching, painting, refibreglassing and restrutting as required. Up on the 'hard', tethered at a marina or sailing the high seas, they go together. He keeps abandoning a comfortable domesticity to go sailing. He won't retire in front of the evening news with a companion to fetch his slippers and keep his bed warm. What propels him forth, even now at the arthritic, muscle-wasting age of seventy-seven? Why is he so restless? What does he expect from this trip? I take his plate. 'I'm going down to rest for a bit. Call me if you need me.'

I try to sound strong and confident but I don't like down below, where yuck feelings float around like thick vomit. He looks up and smiles, then turns his attention to the wind, the sails and back to me.

'We'll need to change the sails soon. I want to take down the storm jib so we can point higher. But have a rest first.'

In my bunk behind the galley, almost on top of the dirty dishes and squashed packets of instant soup, I first push aside clothes, bags and towels to make some room. Fortunately, he calls me back soon. The boat plunges head-first into the swell, spraying a broken sheet of cool water over us both as we take down the storm jib. Dad's not so nimble any more; his eyes make fuzzy images and his reflexes are slow. We work slowly and steadily, dragging the orange mass into the cockpit, then returning to raise the main.

Yesterday, the radar reflector flew into the sea leaving tangled, broken rope way up high. The tangle catches the main halyard that pulls up the main, so it won't go up. Dad doesn't panic when things go wrong, so I don't either. We stay calm. Physical tangles are easy to beat. Step by step we plan what to do and rush down to the cockpit only when a particularly full squall breaks over us. I walk the length of the boat with the end of the halyard and shake. I swing and pulse the rope, snakelike, from my hand to the masthead, from different vantage points. What else can I do?

'Dad, it's free!' I yell. 'We're okay.'

Dad's never been defeated by a tangle. The main halyard whips loose in the wind and catches around the mast steps, tangling us up again. I can't have cleated it off properly. With the little sheet left free, I pull the sail up a bit and then let it down. I send it up and down, hoping for a miracle. The halyard frees up enough for the sail to go up to the first reef, which is all we need for now. Then I wait patiently in the spray while Dad busies himself with new possible solutions. The sun slips down through a misty horizon and the skin of the sea becomes silvery and weathered.

As we clamber back down into the cockpit, Dad turns as if to go back. 'Maybe we'd be safer with the storm gib after all, the wind's coming up.'

'You've got to be joking,' I shout, almost hysterically. 'It's getting dark. We can point higher into the wind now. We don't want to miss Fiji as well.'

I look forward to my night watch. Under the stars and moon, alone in the rugged peaks and deep rolling swells, watching shining walls of wobbly glass collapse into lacy froth, I slip into a subtle place.

When I planted the pencil cross of 'spirituality' on my passage of meaning, the discipline of meditation became the mast on which I raised my sail. For years I followed my breath into subtle experiences of mind. I poked and pushed the boundaries of consciousness; I learned how to break open the shell of 'me' and pour myself out. When I opened my heart, life poured in. I learned to take a truly big breath.

I have been face-to-face with this gorgeous creature *life* many times, and I always lose her and end up shipwrecked on broken stumps of coral. Maybe I set a wrong course or mischievous winds blew me away. I was always sure of my destination: enlightenment. I was certain that from this lofty mountaintop I would make sense of my life. The charts I studied showing the way didn't seem to include the swamps and thickets of ordinary living, so I got confused. Well, I don't have any spiritual charts with me now or spiritual books – I don't trust them. I'm going to head back to where I came from in the beginning, like a homing pigeon, to that place that felt like 'home'. Then I will set out again and this time I'll keep my wits about me.

The wind rises back up to forty knots, piling four-metre swells in front of us. My back is bruised from last night, when I flew into the navigation table, clutching packets of six different flavours of soup for Dad to make a choice. I feel sorry for myself.

'Mum, I need soda water and a cabin bread – now. Pleeaase.'

I do what she asks, without much warmth.

Her pained face fixes me – three motherly things and already you're sick to death of it. You don't know how to be a real mum – and falls back down on her sickbed, tangling up in a blanket of angry memories.

Jack is less flushed and his hands have started roaming. He finds the Weetbix packet in the food cupboard. Flaky biscuit sprays from his dry mouth as he grabs a soft wrinkled carrot from the string hammock in front, leaving the furry tomatoes about to ooze. I'd take them out if I could be bothered.

At the navigation table, with my dividers and pencil, I mark our progress.

'We're still four days away from Fiji. We're holding our course, which is good news, and averaging 100 miles a day, which is bad news.'

Jack utters a long agonised groan. 'It's too long.' He can't fight and he won't surrender.

I take over the watch from Dad. Emily follows me up and falls into my arms, a pathetic bundle of misery. She needs to get away from the lingering smell of sickness and diesel down there. The wet galley floor is stuck with bits of food. We push aside wet discarded clothes, dropped where they were taken off, to make room for our feet. The kitchen sink is full of dirty dishes. I'm tired of being the hero. I'll hunt down a large tin of salmon, a jar of olives and a tomato for lunch.

Our life wasn't always as hard as this. At Orere Point, a gentle paradise by the sea, the soar of seagulls and swallows reminded us to live lightly, but we never really did. Charlotte, then six, sipped crystal dew from nasturtium leaves that hung over the cliff and I turned their seed pods into capers. Emily, twelve, hunted for hen's eggs all over the garden and we turned them into pancakes with lemon and sugar, and Oliver held his honey-soaked hand in front of our hives to feed the starving bees. I had a small car which crossed the beach for seaweed compost. We lived on fruit and nuts, vegetables and shellfish in a garden of Eden.

I remember the pumpkins from Orere.

'Jack, can you get up a minute. I need to get into the food lockers.'

He shuffles over to Emily's bunk as I toss aside his sleeping bag and squab, and disappear head-first into the bowels of the boat, hands groping ahead of me. I can feel them but I can't see them. I finally emerge with my arms full.

'Look, pumpkins. We'll have pumpkin stew for dinner – it'll make us better.'

Emily looks at Jack and they both cringe.

On the floor of the cockpit, soft rain falling, crumpled orange storm-sail in a heap beside me, I attack the thick skin, until juice wells up on the cut surfaces. 'What we need is a good meal. I'll cook it up with coconut milk, ginger and onion.'

Emily smiles and stretches out under the dodger. 'I just threw up again,' she confides. 'Mum, I may go back to Golden Bay. I was happy there with my friends.'

Dream-maker sweeps us through mountainous swells, through squalls and sunshine, night and day. Fierce winds turn her bow and the wind vane drives her back to the course Dad sets.

I stand on deck, face into flying spray, gazing into sparkling jewels and diamonds. Mist, thrown up by the wind, catches the sun. I soar into the light-filled realm of myth and legend, leaving my rain-coated, thermal-undercoated solidity behind. I'm no longer just sailing to Fiji, I am on a holy quest – a simple open-hearted hero in search of her grail.

When I stomp back down the companionway, I have to return to the human realm. When I come out on deck, I return to a light-filled mysterious realm. Where do I belong?

In bed, I keep firmly wedged against the constant motion of the sea. My lee-cloth is useless. Every time I move, and I move a lot, I have to re-position my arms, legs, shoulders and bum against the hull, poking appendages into the corners, making myself rigid on the outside. Howling wind, crashing waves and creakings amplify until it seems like the whole boat is breaking up. Creakings and crackings reverberate inside my head. The inside shell of the boat is slowly separating from the hull. Things throughout the boat rustle and roll. Shards of a beer mug, dashed to a thousand pieces this afternoon, now hide with raisins safely out of sight behind discarded clothes.

'Are you ready for your afternoon story?' I take out my book and settle on Emily's bunk. 'Today, we'll have a short story by Doris Lessing, from her book on the nature of human love.'

Jack tightens his closed eyes. Emily stares at me hopefully.

Then Barbara looked again at Graham, asking silently: All right now, isn't that enough? He could see her eyes, sullen with boredom.

I pick hopelessly through the selection looking for something more uplifting – nothing.

'Poetry might be more inspiring,' I suggest.

'That's a better idea.' Emily looks at Jack, who opens his eyes slightly, then scrunches them even more tightly.

I used to read fairy tales to my children for the spiritual messages tucked up inside. I soared on the golden seams while they drifted off to sleep. I didn't bring any fairy tales.

'I brought a collection of New Zealand poetry.'

Emily's face turns unsure – about the poetry or about siding against Jack?

Time, sweeping, desolates your best hours,
  and your hand stays, short of miracle.

I start another poem. It begins cheerily, but then …

Deep peace! Yet there was terror shut inside;
  And no sound pierced the loneliness, no voices cried.

I'll try again. I flick through the book.

In middle life when the skin slackens
  Its loving clasp of our loose volumes.

I poke inside the book locker for something else.

'I did bring it, a book of Khrishnamurti's commentaries on living. Here we go:

  What is life all about. The sun was beating down on the soft pebbly
  road, and it was pleasant in the shade of the big mango tree.

'The bit at the beginning of each commentary is for warm-ups,' I warn them. 'He'll soon gets down to the nitty-gritty.

  You have all admitted that you are rather confused. Now, do you
  think a confused mind can find out what the purpose of life is?'

Am I a confused mind? I keep reading.

The fact is that whatever a confused mind seeks and finds must also be confused.

This is not helping much.

It's hard to realise because of our conceit. We think we are so clever, so capable of solving human problems.

I give up and put the book down.

In the long silence that follows, the boat's groaning and straining against itself grows into ugly frightening noises. I scream, 'Dad, *Dream-maker*'s about to fall apart. You need to fix the noise.'

He appears in the companionway. 'It's okay, you helped me. The boat wasn't built properly, but I think it'll hold up. I fibreglassed in a couple more struts before we left.' He turns to go back out.

'You've got to be kidding!' I shriek. 'You have to do something.'

He looks at our faces. 'Okay.' We clear out a couple of lockers, so he can inspect his struts. 'One of them has come away. I can screw it back into place – that should stop the noise.'

It doesn't take him long and the noise goes, simple as that. He returns to his watch.

'What a makeshift fix-up job,' Jack mumbles. 'The boat's going to sink with all of us in it.'

My coffin bunk is oppressive. I sink into muscle sliding backwards and forwards across a tether of braced bone, then let my arms and legs roll loose, given up to the sea. The wave-like ebb and flow is not smooth or soothing – it's lumpy and chaotic. A faint smell of diesel pervades. I feel seasick. Dad runs the engine most evenings to recharge our useless batteries. Most times I accept the movement, the noise, the smell and the huge effort required even to boil a cup of water.

Six-thirty every evening we radio into Auckland Cruising. Other boats report in on crew still seriously seasick and distressed. Emily isn't the only person in the universe who's sick. She relaxes. She gets a reprieve from feeling guilty about being such a lame arse; she knows she could do better. Nobody bothers to ask for a forecast. We're still battling 35 to 45 knots head winds even though Auckland Cruising's been telling us for days the winds are reducing to 25 knots.

Outside in the fresh breeze, I snuggle into the collar of my jacket and check our course. Moonlight spills into the dark sea all around. Up in the heavens, sultry clouds hang heavily over the surface of the sea; stars hasten across the sky, like a great tribe crossing vast celestial planes.

M y meditation teachers told me to abandon both thinking and imagination, to cut through all human embellishment and concepts. They encouraged me to burrow deeper than words could follow, down to the ground of being. They said truth was to be found way beneath the sea, not on the surface. From the bottom of the sea, on the inside of my experience, the surface would look different.

My spiritual teachers said that imagination and thinking were near enemies of truth, rather than its friend. Krishnamurti said, 'truth is a pathless land.' I gaze up to the heavens. What am I to do? I can't even get going without conceptual tools. I need imagination to give me a glimmer of what I'm looking for. I need the rudder of rationality, so my boat can keep the course I set. Without thought and imagination my boat would never leave the dock. Is it truth I'm looking for?

I look down at the wake rushing past the hull, shining in moonlight. *Dream-maker* drives steadily through the stormy seas – she seems to know where she's taking us.

3

Eight years ago I experienced the world in a radically different way. A door in my mind opened. I was cycling through the countryside, the wind in every breath, rather like on this sailing trip.

I had been living on the fringe of society for many years, away from the city at a seaside village, Orere Point. I was a serious meditator, yogi and solo mum, happy in the small world of my children and my glorious garden. I had returned without a plan after seven months travelling through south-east Asia and Nepal. Emily, then sixteen, had a new blue mountain bike. I had just enough money to buy one for myself. We crammed a tent, cooker and sleeping bags into our panniers and set out for the coast road between Whitianga and East Cape. That cycling trip changed me forever.

I stagger into the galley with the kettle. I can't face another day in the mess. I'm at the turning point – I'd rather clean up the muck than live in it. This sailing trip will turn into one big clean-up. Of course, big clean-ups create a worse mess in the process. I'm ready for that too.

The morning chorus begins with Emily rolling over to brush away sticky hair and untwist from her blanket. 'Mum, I can only eat when you feed me. Can you feed me some pumpkin soup?'

Does she want me to make up for all the times I was too busy to choo-choo the baked bean train into her mouth or fly the porridge aeroplane into its hangar?

'No, I'm going to clean up this morning. You'll have to feed yourself.'

I remember the day she discarded me. She didn't want to follow my dreams, she didn't want my dreams for her, and she didn't know her own. She's back in that wobbly place now.

I put water on to boil, gather everything from the floor, get down on my hands and knees and scrub. I clean every surface, cubbyhole, plate and fork. I stay centred in the rolling motion, so I won't fall over, practicing for the real thing, life. I keep busy.

Emily sighs and stretches out long, eyes flickering open with boredom. When the last bowl of dirty water has gurgled down the sink, she resumes. 'Mum, can you bring me a drink?'

'Thank you.' She manages a tiny smile. 'Can you peel me a carrot?'

I return the smile. 'They're too soft and wrinkled to peel, but the flavour's concentrated.'

The rain is full and noisy. She will get well, the rain will wash her clean. Clothes flung to the floor, she grabs a cake of soap and clambers up into the cockpit. Dad's out on watch, away from the misery inside, but she doesn't care. I would tell her to make an effort but I won't; I won't threaten our fragile situation.

On our cycling trip, before she discarded me, we flew off forest tracks together and tumbled upside down into the bush, calling out to each other to be rescued. We laughed at every misadventure and hid from storms in mountain huts way off the beaten track. Hills were big and never-ending, but we'd reach the top together, glowing, sharing the last drop of water from our bottles. Cooking up hot lunches on the road-side, snoozing in the shade of tree ferns, we were a team. When she left by bus to go back to school, it was late January. I continued on around the Cape by myself. I sink back down into the memories. It's a good way of not dealing with us now.

The Cape was a landscape of silvery-leaved pohutukawas, stately puriris, rocky coves and dark water. I was cycling in the middle of summer. On big hills, I pushed my bike up through the sticky tar and glowing black jewels, overexposed to the sun, taking too little water, becoming nauseous. Plump, juicy blackberries hanging over the road stewed sweet for breakfasts and dinners. I cycled through wide open spaces, wheels rolling under the steady rhythm of my feet pushing down on the pedals. Caressed by the wind and wild flowers, I followed the sun from dawn till dusk and fell into the huge space around me.

I remember stopping for lunch past the Kereu River, sheltering from the sun in the branches of an old pohutukawa. I bit into a wild peach, plucked from where the snaking Motu River meets the sea. I was all alone, with no one to hold me to the human point of view. The steady turning of wheels had quietened my mind, softened its edges. My mind rested on a hovering sparrow, a flower spray of blue moths fluttering above golden grass, the sparkling, rolling sea. My focus stayed wherever I placed it; it didn't move except to sink into what I was looking at.

I worried about being on my own, even though I wouldn't admit it.

A young Maori fella wandered over to my camp the first night out. He was stoned. 'You're on your own, eh? Would you like one?' He reached his dirty hand into his pocket.

The first few days I imagined Emily with me. In my journal I wrote to her: 'The bread's turned into crumbs but they taste delicious. The honey's run out of the jar and I'm licking it off everything. Your bedroll is soft on the pebbles and I pace myself up the hills by pretending you're in front. I need a swim but you always go in first.'

I wrote: 'The playful breeze lifting my clothes and tickling my body is the same as gentle waves, bubbling the edge of the sand. My veined, wrinkled hand, this driftwood, our past similarly carved into form.' My mind slipped behind what it was looking at, into a soft, clear, intelligent light. The light became seashells and falling leaves in its dance with me. In a direct way I beheld the universe as 'one verse', everything was the same: my hand, the driftwood, the gentle waves – the same. It didn't seem strange; it seemed natural, obvious. Emily disappeared and I became contented in a way I had never known.

Then I slipped further away, behind the soft intelligent light that turned into seagulls, back behind to a place that held the very possibility of perception – the very possibility of experience – as a miracle. I stood on the beach and looked at the seagulls. We were all suspended in space; this space was suspended in mind, unfathomable mind, where perception is the magician's wand. I had no idea how a universe could possibly arise from this place, but it did. It was as if a magician waved a wand and the world rabbit appeared from the void, moment by moment. The seagull was renewed with every wave of the wand, every moment of perception.

I saw that perception, which I had always taken for granted, was a most extraordinary phenomenon. Perception brings a world to life. Perception creates something out of nothing, the actual out of potential. Mind, moment by moment, constructs seagulls, driftwood, me and the mercurial sea.

I walked slowly back across the sand as my mind gathered itself back into my body. Everything around me was as it had been before. Campers were eating at plastic tables, clipped open, not far from their cars. Seagulls faced into the wind like sentries. I watched the sun sink below far tree-scaped hills. The sea turned orange; its sparkles disappeared. The fading light dressed the sea in an evening gown of slinky, wrinkled velvet and then the water turned grey. Seagulls cried, swell broke on the shore. I walked to my tent and snuggled down into my feathery sleeping bag. I felt so safe on the ground. There was nowhere to fall.

There's still a long way for us to fall on the boat. Emily finishes dancing in the rain and returns to her sick bed, glancing at Jack, who doesn't look up, closing back into herself.

I go out to sit with Dad and pretend its all okay. He's over it. 'I'll never go sailing with Emily and Jack again. I've never had such useless crew.'

He stares out to sea, clamping up inside himself, glancing across to me. The rigging on the mizzen jangles uselessly.

'Dad, they're sick. You know Emily's not like this.'

'I've never had to put up with such uselessness. Good crew will their seasickness away.' His crossed legs quiver and start his feet kicking up.

I start to nod in agreement, but change direction. He's the enemy. 'Crew on the other boats are still very seasick. We haven't had a break.'

'Jack should never have come. I could tell at the Barrier that he wanted to leave. I should have encouraged him to go.'

'Emily may have gone as well.'

He stomps away to his hole behind the navigation table to disappear inside headphones. I check the compass to make sure we're on course, then check the arrow at the top of the mast for the wind direction and the angle of the waves for confirmation, and finally the set of the sail for signs of useless flapping. This gives me a clear picture of our situation.

I'm her mother, what does he expect. I'm easily confused by currents and winds. I stomp back and forth in the cockpit wanting everything to be different. I check the sails again and the wind vane, to see if anything's changed.

A few years ago Emily and I were caught out in a mountain storm. She was tough, and walked in front with the heavier pack. This seasickness is something else. I should tell them to make lunch. They need to want to be well. Why don't they? What's wrong with 'well'? My courage to confront them fails. It's not up to me.

At least the outside storm has finished and our wet dirty clothes are airing in the cockpit, soaking up sunshine. I want us all to be happy. I'll cook Orere eggs for dinner, for their red healing yokes. In the shade of the dodger, I drift back to my cycling trip. Then, I had all the answers.

I slept on a different beach every night and always packed early to get over the hills before the heat. One morning I was sanding my dishes clean in a stream, when a fellow camper enquired, 'Do you like crayfish?'

I looked up into the face of a friendly camper. 'I love crayfish!'

I had forgotten how to speak until I started and then I couldn't stop. I wanted to share my adventures and stories; I wanted to say how amazing life was that I should be sharing crayfish with them in their tent. The sun was climbing. I packed a crayfish and six paua into my panniers for later, swung my leg over onto my bike and waved like a soaring gull. I pedalled off into the miraculous. Their truck stopped at the bottom of the next hill, so I threw my bike into the back and flew with them to the summit, face into the wind. The whole of life was an extraordinary outpouring of generosity.

Summer was as long as forever, cycling into Waihau Bay. On a dusty gravel road, a local store, pumping gas and selling bread. My legs hung over the jetty with my tongue curled around a boysenberry ice cream. Childhood was as close as the sprats swimming around the slimy poles. I stared into pure blue water and poked at limpets and barnacles. I found the mind I was before words claimed it for someone else's story. The child mind of wonder is creamy, uncurdled custard before language reheats it into lumpy stodge.

I pedalled on around the top of the cape, into marginal farm country full of ragwort, blackberry and flowering gorse. Scrawny animals browsed between the weeds and kahikatea. At the Oweka stream I splashed in the cool water, blinking salty sweat from my eyes, then feasted on crayfish, leaving the carcass for the blowflies. Sunk in long grass, warm breeze caressing my face, I let the bubbling stream trickle through my empty body.

I wondered about time and memory, concepts that hadn't troubled me before. I had used the words like everyone else, without thinking. Now they rose up like signposts, big words, telling me something about myself. Cycling day after day into the present, I realised I was losing my familiar sense of 'me'. Lying next to this trickling stream, I watched my mind flicker away into past and future, drawing on memory to keep 'me' alive.

I remembered painting the walls of my home, helping Emily with her history exam, snuggling up to Charlotte. I got the scary inkling that I only existed as these memories. I watched the images pass by: being absorbed in the flow of Tai Chi, digging potatoes from my garden, coaxing school children into headstands and complicated yogic poses. This was 'me' in the realm of time. Without these memories I didn't exist. I didn't want to exist.

I sat up, so I could think more clearly. Memory and time were mental, they weren't in the world. I was onto something. Obviously, if 'I' was the work of my mind, so was my world. For some reason I was desperate to slip away from myself, my memories, the ones that constructed a 'me.'

Sitting in the long grass, unhinged from these memories, absorbed in the beauty of the afternoon, I became perplexed. I couldn't see any reason to do anything. It was only the past that pointed the finger and presented the dilemmas of choice. It was my past that asked the questions and grew pictures for me to live. What if I could abandon my past?

I cycled around to Hicks Bay in the cool afternoon, all the way along to a large jetty right down the end. Big ships must have come in here once. I stepped into the spell of pickled wood and flaking iron, sea and sun, barnacles and silvery sprats, beginnings and endings of journeys. As a child I used to hang out on jetties and wonder. I was one big question mark.

The next morning I wandered down to the beach. Without language tugging my skirts, I wasn't fixed as anything in particular. A sense of lighthearted play, a delight in just being, carried me over the sand. The sun conjured vast shadowy landscapes from the sand and stone.

When my children were young, we played landscape games. Emily took huge leaps from mountaintop to mountaintop, crossing braided river plains, laughing to make this other world real, happy because she knew her way back to me. At Hicks Bay I looked down into moonscape craters and broad rocky mountain ranges. Sandy cliffs sprouted yellow grass and green hills rolled into the forest. Were they a hundred metres high, great towering sandy bluffs, or ordinary-sized banks? I couldn't tell by looking. Were the breaking waves nature's fury or playful rolling tongues at the water's edge? Imagination or reality?

A mighty seagull strutted across the sand, warning me away with its sharp eyes, brilliant red beak and stick legs; it was defending the tides. When the breeze ruffled its feathers and distinguished air, it paddled away. I paddled away too, along a gravel road, through clouds of yellow fennel pollen to a grassy knoll beaded with dew. In another bay, fluffy white clouds reflected in the sand, the tide remaking the mirror-like surface in big sweeping arcs. A tractor, silvery vessel in tow, chortled down to the sea and the beach filled with three children – six if you counted their reflections – shorts held up as they giggled in the frothy foam. The sun reminded me of the day ahead and I hurried away to pack.

4

I'm learning everything I can about sailing. I read about practical things like hypothermia, Danforth and CQR anchors, starboard and port lights, drogues. I read about emergency signalling and the difference between VHF (very high frequency) and SSB (single side band) radios. VHF is used for line of sight communication and SSB, which bounces off the ionosphere, is used to send messages across larger distances. We use SSB to communicate with Auckland Cruising back in New Zealand and will use VHF to get in touch with customs when we arrive in Suva.

I focus in on the secret detail of anchor weight and shape. I'm a good student, it was my life raft. I learned how to dive eagerly into anything that wasn't me, turtle-back protection, head in front keeping my heart safe, bright sharp lights in my head, dark shadows everywhere else. I used textbooks for my templates of life and 'A's on report cards for my rites of passage. I don't care much for this creature now. It hides away from the mystery. It can't even approach questions about truth or meaning.

The wiry, sunburnt sailing animal in me enjoys living. It lives from memories lurking way beneath words and a human story. It grew from an intelligence far greater than the one I use to study and philosophise and analyse things. I'm depending on it.

Jack's face has some colour, and his limbs move with more intent. He's still horizontal on his bed, counting down the days, forward focus; he will get to live and be in control again. He won't ever go to sea again. Emily still insists on throwing up, even though the seas are calm. Together they venture outside and creep into the shade of the sail up on deck, to look on the vast ocean and resurrect their relationship. Jack drones a steady deep monotone. Emily flutters and warbles around him.

'Mum, I need you to cook me some rice and get me something to drink.'

Dad rushes to my rescue. 'How are you this morning, Alice? Would you like me to make you a cup of tea?'

I mutter almost incoherently, 'I'm fine,' and start cooking the rice, tossing pots and lids to find the courage. 'Emily, I want you and Jack to do the dishes.'

'We aren't well,' she retorts back through the hatch.

'I don't care. I want you to do them.' I turn the rice down so it doesn't boil up all over the stove and floor.

The hours pass, and the dancing voices rise and fall above me. When I start the dishes Jack comes down. 'We were waiting until it was cool.'

Dad hangs the black solar shower from the mizzen boom and strips for his first shave and shower since leaving New Zealand. His voice blossoms into a normal cheery. 'Alice come and have a shower. It'll do you good.'

I'm too black inside, like the hanging bag of water. I try for cheery but end up in dull and heavy. 'I need to rest. I'll shower later.'

Stretched out on Emily's sickbed under a breeze wafting through the open hatch, I remember the parts of sailing that don't have Emily and Ted in them. I took the last reef out of the main all by myself this morning. Last night Dad took a sleeping pill, confident I could reduce the headsail on my own if the wind came up. This morning, with a drawing, he explained clearly how the batteries, power switches and charging work. I understood.

He comes down to Emily's sickbed for a chat. 'Jack's got a lot of growing up to do.' He folds into his belly, face intent, eyes scanning the cupboards across the saloon. 'Young people today have gone soft on it. In my day, I had to milk a dozen cows in the dark before I walked to school, barefooted, for miles every day.'

I sit up grimacing, clamping up inside. I don't want to hear this. I know how hard it was in his day.

'Dad, the challenges are different today.' I won't let him rubbish Emily. 'Kids have emotional issues to sort out, more than physical ones.'

'I haven't seen much emotional maturity from Jack or Emily.'

'I know.'

'The physically robust quality is missing in their generation.'

'Yes, it is.'

Dad's very interested in metaphysics. I steer in a different direction, once he has a warm beer in his hand, so we can stay close.

'We're both interested in the nature of our minds. I want to talk about the things I've discovered through meditation. Are you interested?'

'Sure, I won't interrupt.' He relaxes.

I start out in a way I have never done before with anyone – to clear the air, to join us back together, to prove myself worthy of his love, to justify my existence to him – for all sorts of tortured reasons.

'When my mind is soft and clear and my heart is very open, I sometimes find that my sense of self, which is ordinarily wrapped up in my thoughts and desires, shifts to the outside world. I become identified with everything outside of me. The outside world becomes me. I don't exist inside myself anymore. There is no inside. My mind is the space around me and everything in it is made of this space-mind-stuff. What is most exciting is that this space-mind seems intelligent, conscious and creative. I am this mind-stuff. I'm the dream-maker dreaming the world.'

'Ahha. By dreaming this world you mean you are creating your own reality?'

Dad finishes his beer and drops the bottle to the floor with a clatter. I produce a tin of salted peanuts.

I sit with my legs crossed, to focus us, keep our minds sharp. 'Well, not exactly. I don't control this dreaming. I'm not sure anyone controls it. Maybe this mind-stuff is the creative fermenting of life. When my sense of self is attached to this mind-stuff, the dualistic world of 'you' and 'me' is transcended – you're right – and I see myself as the creator I truly am. The problem is the little 'self' that is so interested in creating a world to suit itself no longer exists.'

I turn into his gaze with the sting. 'This is where you and I part company. There is no creator separate from the whole of life. Being separated out is the illusion, the illusion that creates suffering.'

Dad recoils like clockwork. 'Yes, it's just as I thought, you Buddhists want to deny life.'

He stands up, to sweep his arm wide. 'Look around you. We live in a wonderful world. We're meant to enjoy it.'

'I agree.' I recoil like clockwork and we are back in our same old roles. 'Buddhism isn't negative. My life is much richer when I reach beyond the illusion of being trapped inside myself.'

'We are limited by our thoughts. Ramtha says limitless thought leads to limitless life. Life will give you what you expect.'

Dream-maker lurches over a wave, rights herself, and speeds onwards through the wind, keeping the angle set by the wind vane.

'Dad, that's not true. You can't fly just because you think you can. The thought that built you into a human being is not a thought you can change.' My mind races in lots of directions. 'Maybe if you studied for years in the Himalayas you could learn to fly.'

'Exactly.'

We're in trouble. Our views don't match, but they almost do and so we fudge the edges and slide into nonsense. I need a point of view to have a discussion, I need to fit experience into concepts to have a discussion, I'm losing the plot completely, I always do with him.

I try again for reasons I don't understand. 'I agree that the small ordinary mind we live in creates its reality to some degree. It separates out a 'self' and, within limits, creates according to the desires and fears of this 'self'. But this little 'self' is not necessarily

in charge of its desires. Did you create your desire for romance?
Maybe it was created thousands of years ago and is just using you
to stay alive. There's no way you can stop getting old, however
much you wish and scream. The dreamer who fixed death into
your genes is much more powerful than you. Where did your desire
to go sailing come from? Did you think it up all on your own?'

'If I really believed I wasn't going to get old, I wouldn't,' he
retorts. 'The trouble is everyone around me believes I'm getting
old. That's why I don't tell anyone my age. If I did they would
treat me differently. I've read of people in the Himalayas who
have never died.'

'Well, Dad, I guess I'm not interested in using the power of
thought to change my circumstances or escape death, but rather
to understand life. I want to know, just to know, to solve the
puzzle of who I am and why I am here. I guess we're interested in
spirituality for different reasons.'

'Yes, maybe we are. Life is a miracle. The older I get the more
I appreciate this.'

I get up to make us a cup of tea. I don't understand why I get
so angry, why I have to nail him, persuade him. He brought me
up to fight like this. I let him talk as he wants now, until he leaves
to take over the watch from Emily and Jack.

'Mum, you can stay on my bunk, I'll rest with Jack.'

Their thin bodies curl up together as they drift off to sleep.

Cycling around East Cape I was without these mental
gymnastics. I had only one mind to deal with and it was
quieting down in the rhythm of cycling and the constant physical
exertion. I turned the pedals over and over, hour after hour,
day after day. I cycled up the hill and then down into another
desolate bay. I followed the steady whirr of tyres on soft tarmac,
as they rolled past bulrushes, stands of manuka, clearings of
grass and yellow maize, brick chimneys, crooked wee shacks
with fresh washing strung into the wind. I fell in love, dissolving
into the flowering grasses, marshes, cicadas, seagulls, gazing in

wonder at the textures, colours and patterns until I was nothing but this beauty.

I didn't stop until I came to the Waiapu River, where I pitched my tent on her parched, mud-crusted banks. Dust had turned the river grey and the dust-filled air was hard to breathe. Paradise ducks welcomed me as the only other sign of life – straggly gorse bushes and the occasional blowfly don't count. I lay down, sticky and dusty, too tired to care. When I asked for water and directions earlier, the headmaster of a local school invited me to stay at the school. I could have camped under shady trees with water and electricity nearby but my human skin doesn't fit so well – it never has. I was looking for a way to grow a new one, even though I didn't understand this at the time. I continued along the lonely gravel road to its end, over smelly swamps, across marginal farmland where battered cars lay abandoned and careless fires scarred the gorse – a skeleton among skeletons, finally at rest in my bones.

It was afternoon before I washed my face and limbs in a little precious bottled water and went exploring. Piles of smooth white tree skeletons, washed ashore by the dark, steeply rolling, unfriendly sea, stretched along the whole beach. I set about climbing over and around them along the beach, finally turning back to the river's mouth, shining now in the setting sun. A fine misty light softened the trees, gold water licked small stones and I melted back into the bosom of the sweetest mother.

Morning sun poured in through the mosquito netting. A young lad had arrived to check his fishing net. I'd been cycling for three weeks and I needed a break. The shade of the gorse was cool now, but the sun was rising, bringing the heat, so I had to keep moving.

A squashed possum appeared on the road, its unbroken ribcage poking out through a bloody, hairy carcass. I suddenly realised, in a brand new way, that our ribcages were the same. I had dissected many animals at university. I had known since then that we were the same, in an ordinary kind of way. I never recognised what it implied, we were the same! Grown from the same intelligence. From that glimpse I gained a dead-sure sense that I was onto something. Other people and I were the same as well, the same as in identical, behind our superficial faces. Whatever song was singing us, it was the same one. We were the same tune in an awesome symphony. My mind had pulled us apart. I wanted to keep us together: the possum, me, other people. We were the same. This was the truth. I didn't doubt it for an instant and yet to live this truth, to act from this truth, how was that going to be possible? I knew that it would take a very different person from me to live this truth.

I rested on the silty bank of the Mangaopara River. Poplar trees shivered in the wind. I was cycling into a great vortex of living that kept opening out, like the spiral heart of the flowers. No words to fix the experience. Life was unspeakably magnificent and totally unfathomable – parading a quality of awesome power. Images from the fairy stories I read my children flickered through my mind – mountains opening up into underground caverns filled with jewels, dogs with eyes like saucers. These stories described this ungraspable prescience. I didn't understand what I was cycling into, I only knew it was real and there was nothing I could do with it.

By the time I passed the Ruatoria turnoff, I was done pedalling. Hunger, tiredness and thirst tugged incessantly, like young children pulling at my shorts, so I disembarked in the tidy garden of a school, under a spreading plane tree, tipping the food pannier out into its litter of bark and cones. My eyes, soon close to horizontal, focused onto the cones growing their own gardens of lichen and moss, hosting even smaller gardens, on and on forever inwards and outwards into the grand trees and beyond.

An hour later the cool wind stroked my bare arms awake. Weak and unsteady, I staggered to my feet, spitting thick phlegm, and wandered back to the toilets. Undressed over a child-sized sink with my cake of soap for a wash, I couldn't decide what to do next. I was worn out but I didn't know how to not keep going. Under the plane tree I gazed up through unhurried leaves, settled into the earth underneath, and filled with a deep contentment. I would go on. My bicycle was taking me somewhere, just like *Dream-maker*. It had plans I knew nothing about.

My off-road tyres gripped well on the rough gravel road that plunged steeply down to the coast. I flew past painted fences, flower gardens and brick paths. I passed the prettiest homesteads of the entire trip. The campsite on Waipiro beach was disappointing though; wire strings enclosed rusting caravans, long grass and rubbish. On the beach, a young father was trying to get his five very young children into a van. They fluttered, in brightly coloured skirts and shirts, far from his outstretched arms. The fishing rods and boxes waited in the back without any fuss. He suggested another campsite further along.

I arrived without water, to find the river grey with silt. Emily and I had waited this cyclone out in a forest hut a week ago. Swinging empty water containers, I walked back to the local boat club where an annual fishing contest was in full swing. Farmers and fishermen – ruddy leathered faces – thick swollen hands, talked in deep, slow, familiar ways about their lives. This could my father's family – people of the land and sea. Children frisked in the long grass, stepping crabwise over the rocks to plunge into the crashing waves. They spilled in and out of adult conversation, squeezing tomato sauce over sausages cradled in white bread, pouring fizzy drink into plastic cups. I had a childhood like this.

Next morning under an overcast sky, I made my way up a tumbling stream, crossing and re-crossing the slippery stones. I scrambled onto a large rock. Ants scurried in and out of one crack; quartz crystals grew out of another. The ants scurried over me. They were manoeuvering a grass seed into the crack. My mind started pouring into what I was looking at; it slipped totally away from me. I became what I was seeing. The boundaries keeping me separate from the ants disappeared. I became the rocks and ants and grass seed. I became what I was looking at. I slipped right inside, underneath the surface, and discovered pure love. It felt like sweet milky melted marshmallows. Back and forth I went. I drew my mind back inside my body, separate from the ants and grass seed and then I let it go. I realised this mystical at-one-ment is the way it was for all of us, way back in the beginning before thought and language and disappointment took us away.

I am the sea that roars and cries and falls silent
I know, I am, the sea is ME.
I journey back to the beginning of time
still a seed unsprouted.
Hard to imagine now the mighty
hard-headed, hard-eyed goliath it becomes.

I revisit my childhood
when it isn't an issue, blue moths or me
There is only one dancer, that dancer is ME.
I danced as a child, I danced as a moth,
green fields below, blue sky above
I danced them all into life.

Somewhere along the way the music changed
I was left standing watching the dance pass by
Forgetting, forgotten, the dance had gone.

The sound of the river filled the valley. I pulled its song from the cacophonous din of cicadas. The whitish froth of the river's tumble struggled up from the silted water to meet the sun sparkling in the bubbles. The stubborn rocks caused the tumble, made possible the delightful melody and bewitching braids. Rocks turn the stream of life into music! When I was a child, I couldn't understand why outer space was dark and cold when sunlight shone all the way through? My Dad explained: 'Heat and light only appear when something stops the rays, otherwise the light just flies on through.'

Strange how what you've been looking at influences what you see next. In the shade of the manuka on a golden hillside, I gazed the sticky grey riverbed into the clouds – same colour, texture and feeling.

Dandelions wafted by, clouds grew into vast light-filled landscapes and rocks in the bay stood firm against the crashing swell.

How did I come to such a dream? How did I come to be such a dream-maker? I had no idea. All I knew was that I was much more than I ever thought. My body was a rock in a stream of possibility, a planet stopping the rays of the sun. I turned nothing into something. I belonged to life waking up in me. I was a miracle. Why was I so hung up on my own petty life? Why should I struggle to prove myself of value? What a joke! I was incredible without doing anything.

On the hillside, I dreamed dandelions into life and then forgot how to ride with them. How did this happen? I stared the villain, time, into view.

In time I grow a past and future. I cut eternity into pieces for discussion. Time's friend, expectancy, rushes carelessly ahead, trampling truth. In time I am determined, like cloud condensing in the sky, a grain of sand seen separately, a splinter in the eye.

Why did I have to live in the world of time? Why did I have to live with a past and future? I had set out on the path of 'wakening up,' but I didn't know what this meant. I thought it meant waking up from a little 'me' in time into a big eternal 'ME'. If so, what did time have to do with anything? Surely I was finished with it. I just couldn't get where to go to from here.

5

Dream-maker is dedicated to her cargo of misery: Jack trapped inside bubbles of discontent, Emily wafting like a sullen ghost, both shipwrecked from life. They don't know how to get back to the mother ship, to put their feet down on something solid and feel how it will hold them up.

Instead of making lunch, I go outside for fresh air under a clear blue sky, to write in my journal. Jack and Emily hang out on deck, as far away from us as they can get. Every few days a passing bird stops on the mast, and very occasionally a small flying fish strands itself. We haven't seen another boat the whole trip. The days slip by into the sea; I seem to be slipping after them.

Curled up in the corner of the cockpit, I gaze out so that space itself comes into focus, and *Dream-maker* transforms into a light image floating in clear consciousness. I have separated out from myself into a larger view. I turn my gaze back into the insubstantiality of my dream of me, earnestly and seriously writing my journal in a corner of light. I see into the 'me' who believes herself solid, of real substance, who believes her actions are her own, of consequence. I see into her frantic scribbling, determined to keep her dissolution at bay. I see how she writes herself into permanence. She is nothing but the play of form, ignited with a flickering, trembling flame of consciousness that expands into a giant glowing orb holding her in an awesome, compassionate knowing that she, the scribbler, cannot see. I am dreaming my life without realising that I am the dreamer. Only when my consciousness dissolves into this sea of luminous knowing, do I remember I am this boat carrying its crew across the lonely sea.

I let my mind contract again until the boat becomes solid. A wave of nausea passes. I am not ready to get up and slice onions. My mind falls open again. It's a shifting dimension, with breathing and posture changes – as if I'm waking up with a jolt, like an elevator stop – and then I'm suddenly perceiving everything as light, as mind, and I know this view is more real than my ordinary view. I don't know why, I just know. Time is gone, so is thinking, so is my personal story. Love is everywhere, and a quality of knowing everything, of being everything. I am everything and nothing at all. This is what I discovered on my cycling trip.

Everyone's hungry because it's after two. Jack clambers down into the cockpit to get Emily's fluffy grey jacket. The wind is rising. I look up to discover that I'm looking out through his eyes. There is no distinction between him and me. My breath is breathing my dream of him. He doesn't exist for me outside my dreaming. I hear Emily's calling as my dreaming of her. Now he's well enough, Jack is certain of his view. He plans to make money. His voice flows like a knotted rope. Forget the great ocean carrying us on her back – he will stay on land and steer his own course. I admire his naivety.

I get up to throw some pasta into boiling water, open a tin of tuna and chunky tomato pieces and grate some cheese. Emily and Jack wash the dishes afterwards. We're back together.

This time I wriggle with pleasure under warm water sprinkling from our black plastic shower. Emily soaps my back, soothing tired muscles with her strong fingers, tickling around my waist until I flick her with water. She hands me a towel, then sings while I cook dinner and helps pass the food up into the cockpit.

'Mum, this is the first time we've all eaten together.'

'So it is. Maybe we should have done it earlier.' I turn to Dad.

'We're almost there. Why don't you tell us something about Fiji; I don't know anything.'

He puts down his fork. 'Your lack of interest in world affairs has always surprised me. I'm glad to see a change of heart.'

I don't take his comment as a criticism. I've been busy exploring finer realms.

'When the British took over Fiji in the late 1800s, they developed the sugar cane plantations and brought in Indians as indentured workers. The Indians had to work on the plantations for ten years for very little money. After that they could go home or stay and lease land of their own. Nearly half the population is Indian now and they tend to be the businessmen, doctors, lawyers and teachers.'

I'm always surprised how much my father knows.

'Wasn't there a coup a while back?' I ask.

'Yes. Ever since Fiji became independent and democratic in 1970, there have been coups. The army is dominated by Fijians who believe the power of government belongs to the chiefs. When the Indians formed a majority in the government, the army rose up and gave the power back to the Fijians. After the latest coup in 2000 there were reprisals against the Indians. When their leases came up for renewal, their land was taken and given to Fijians. The Fijians claim the Indians hadn't paid their leases. I don't know the full story.'

Jack slips away to the far corner of the cockpit and stares blankly into the sea, willing the seabird with its olive branch, not interested. I start the first watch of the evening. Stars poke through the darkening cloud, lighting up the rest of my cycling trip.

At Waipoi the moon rose soft and full, through pastel pinks and oranges tossed from the dying sun. The sea was tranquil, as if in awe of such a wondrous sight. Sharp bushy-headed rushes stood to attention. She rose slowly through one windswept, sun-soaked cloud bank after another, hidden, only to reappear mysteriously out of the shadows, her glory increasing with the clouds' fade to grey and the sky's deepening blue. Unquestioned ruler of the night she rose, majestic, whole, and her radiance spread across the darkening water. She called me to the wholeness in myself. She spoke of cycles completing themselves. I was spellbound and I didn't know why. She shone down on me cocooned inside my tent, watching baby cockroaches scurry along the zippers and daddy-long-leg spiders climbing up the corners.

At Tolaga Bay I set out on foot to explore, even though I was too tired to soar with the gulls. Shivering rabbit's tails wooed me uselessly.

The extra-long jetty looked like it had been made by nature: the long spinal column of something prehistoric. I imagined people gasping, 'Was I like this, way back then?' It was broken tar seal, with a railway line rusting down to where couples held empty fishing lines in the water. The soft yellow cliffs, beautifully sculptured from their time under the sea and now by wind and water, seemed ordinary to my dull mind.

The next morning I walked across to Cooks Cove, leaving a dark green trail in the dewy grass. I was well-rested and very calm. My mind started expanding all by itself, until it was vast and all-encompassing. And then it changed; it went further than I could follow; it became void – neither dark nor light; it became the boundless empty space of the universe. This mind held a miracle, a hovering glistening bubble of life. The vision was steady, the whole of life hovered. I was holding the universe in the palm of my hand. It stayed a long time – minutes. I had reached back as far as the human mind could go. This was the immaculate conception, our precious bubble of life, the virgin birth. I saw the whole of life spontaneously arising out of nothing:

Bounded bubble of life
Immaculately conceived in a virgin mind
The greatest mystery of them all
This universe floating in space.

Familiarity turned extra-ordinary an ordinary grey.
Busyness and laziness became my way
to hide the shame of my most human fall of all.

Once I looked straight into the face of grace
Too young to hold a past or future
Too young to covet a form
Too young to know the difference.

Now trapped inside, I stand to see what life has done
Euphoria and doubt build me up and tumble me down
Rewritten memories and life's masks,
'Yes please's and 'no thank you's,
They push and pull and dazzle and confuse.

Can I stand without a sound, without a fall?
Present at life's birth, present at its death,
arising and dissolving, moment by moment.

I walked on down to the cove. Cook's ships anchored here when his men came ashore to gather supplies of wood and water. They were adventurers, like me, exploring because it is in our nature to explore.

It was raining when I cycled into Gisborne. The motor camp had big stainless tables for cooking and eating. Barbed wire netting marched around the perimeter, keeping some of us in and others of us out. Noisy bulldozers piled up the storm's debris. I was lost. I wandered the port, the beaches and streets – a homeless soul, not belonging. Georgie Pie was a place to get out of the rain, with pop music playing, jogging my mind. My surroundings had changed from tumbling grass dunes to bright plastic fare but I relaxed into my chair and picked at my pie. In that moment I broke open. I slipped inside everyone eating their pies. I spread way on out and there was that heart again, holding us all in the palm of its hand.

I walked back through the rain, streaming down my face into tears. When the truth appears there never is a doubt. My heart was singing all the way to my tent. When the rain stopped, I opened the fly into the sun pouring down all over me, sunlight coursing through my veins, the energy of my life. I felt blessed. Moments like these, they come and they go. What I would give not to forget that the laws building you, from the smallest cell to the grandest idea, are building me too. We are the same, you and I. I always forget what the important things are.

I bused home from Gisborne with my jewels of truth, and didn't know what to do with them. My children wanted a city life and I was finished with searching. I had found what I was looking for. I fell back through the jaws of time. I drove through heavy traffic every morning, dealt with work problems all day, was a mother for my daughters and two home-stays in the evenings, finished building my new house in the weekends, and wondered if I would ever have enough money to pay the mortgage. I fell heavily from grace into an ordinary person. My jewels turned back into dusty stones I didn't have time to polish.

I haul the main all the way up, mostly by hand, then let off the furling line so the headsail can blow out a little, for a bit more wind. We're still on a tight reach. The main sheet could be loosened a bit as well. We're still heading up as far as we can, on the same tack, in the same wind, the whole trip. Our sails do look beautiful, wide open in the fresh breeze. Light cloud puffs the horizon, sun dances in the water. I love working up on deck with my feet solidly planted on the wobbling platform, limbs bared to the salty air. Pulling up the main, gazing into the boundless sky, I become absorbed in the wondrous miracle that living is. Then Dad calls and I have to shrink back inside my body and scramble into the cockpit to pull in the jib. We chat. The very language we use to talk and bond separates us out, and pulls me away from my great ocean home.

I am discouraged about ending up stuck in this dilemma again and I knew this would be my starting point. An ordinary, uninspired life is an empty delusion, but grasping after the mystical, hunting down eternity, is no life either. Can I even imagine what a synthesis of the mystical and ordinary would look like? Where do heaven and earth meet? I am the magician calling forth a world, so I can drown in its sorrows and joys. What for? Is it possible to wash dishes and talk, knowing I am the dishes and the person drying them? I throw down my journal; I can't imagine an answer and yet there must be one.

I return to the galley to heat up a pot of apparently solid, incontestably nutritious, pumpkin soup. Cupfuls of steaming thick puree pass into the cockpit, followed by crackers and cheese and then me. 'I estimate that we are only twenty-four hours from Suva.'

Even Jack can't help smiling.

'Well guys, what do you think?' I tease. 'Were we brave or stupid. *Dream-maker* hadn't been to sea in three years. She and Dad were retired.'

'Don't be stupid, Mum,' Emily glares. 'We wouldn't have left at all if we'd had a trial sail!'

Dad grinds his teeth. Jack stares out to sea, at freedom just over the next wave.

The night before we arrive I have a dream. I am at Orere Point, with my soul weaving through its leaves and flying out across the ocean view. In my dream, branches of a large pear tree I planted long ago fall down. I am hot and shaking uncontrollably because I'm going to die. My terror of death forces out a cry for help. A neighbour from across the road, who is having a party, helps me to his home. I sit numb and unresponsive in the group of strangers until a particular song is played. Then I rise as if in a trance and begin to dance, very expressively. This happens twice. I return to the street. The whole tree has fallen over. Death approaches. The last thing I have to do is clear away the branches. I make a start. All the branches that grew from my young plant have to be cleared away.

The scene changes. I'm at university and I've missed all my English and French classes, because something very important is happening. Up on the cliff nearby I have a new baby and I go into a small dark alcove to breast feed it. It's well wrapped up and seems calm and content.

I sit down with a friend, in a group of friends, on a rocky promontory overlooking the sea. My friend says firmly and kindly, 'It's time for us to go together.' We lean forward. She pushes me. I fall into the sea, then look up to see her still sitting on the cliff. She has betrayed me. It doesn't matter – I accept I had to go alone. The choppy sea is warm and embraces me like a lover. I drift away, all alone. I will die peacefully, without a struggle. I wake softly into a warm light radiating from my heart.

We approach Suva in the dark. 'I don't understand why the batteries are so flat,' Dad frets. 'What if they won't start the engine when we turn into the harbour? Maybe we should go straight in tonight?'

'I don't think so,' I quickly reply. Dad's way too agitated. 'We haven't sailed using waypoints. Now's not the time to practice.'

'I'll have to keep the engine going all night, then.' I jump when the engine suddenly starts roaring. Dad stays calm. 'The throttle's come adrift. It's done this before. You'll have to go into the engine compartment to fix it. I can tell you what to do.'

Spanner and torch in tow, I elbow in through a small hole under the companionway and fumble around. The two pieces lock back together, noise stops, job done.

'We need to slow the boat down ... ' Dad paces the cockpit in a buzz of confusion. 'Otherwise we'll arrive in the dark.' I reef the main. 'We're still going too fast.' I reef it again and furl most of the headsail.

With the engine running, the inside of the boat is hot and noisy. The lights are off because we need good night sight. I make out shadows of land and white surf breaking over coral.

'You'll have to take all the sail down. We'll stand off until light.'

We bustle around the sleeping bodies of Emily and Jack, over and around wet dirty clothes dropped where they were taken off. The mess is unnerving. I use torch light to read the GPS and plot our approach. We look for definition in the shadows. Dad is becoming increasingly agitated. He doesn't take his high blood pressure medication regularly. I can't suggest anything. We trace and retrace a path a safe distance from the entrance. Getting safely into a harbour is obviously the difficult part of sailing. Dad's breath stays short and hard all night. 'Our boat is jinxed; we've had too many problems; I don't like it,' he grumbles.

'I'll make us a cup of hot soup.'

Dawn wakes up the coastline and we motor safely through the entrance, past the skeleton shipwreck and a motley collection of boats, to a place near shore. We have finally arrived, thirteen wobbly days behind us. Emily and Jack wake up and gaze sleepily around. I remember my dream: clearing branches, a young baby, death and the warm embrace of the ocean.

PART TWO

6

With a yellow quarantine flag tied onto the starboard main stay, I haul the anchor out of the for'ard bunk. Dad creeps into the chain locker and pokes the end of the anchor chain up through the hawsepipe so I can shackle the corroded galvanised link onto the rusty anchor and drop the whole bundle into the harbour. We're here to stay.

The harbour is big, with misty green hills way around the other side – hills as softly romantic in the hazy morning light as the sprawling wharf is harsh with commerce. The angry sound of steel being smashed and beaten into new forms is our new song, the deep-throated rumble of ocean-going liners and smaller container ships its rhythm. A siren reminds me of rigidly punctuated, ordinary working lives – maybe comfortably so. Scruffy yachts and old fishing boats float disinterestedly around us. A breeze carries the fetid smell of garbage, rotting down to compost, from a nearby dump. What a welcome!

Dad gives up control, now the outside pressure is off.

'What's the computer doing on the floor?' he barks. 'Why didn't you pick it up?'

He lifts it from its pool of stale beer and plants it on the front berth.

I retaliate. 'But Dad, you knew it was there. I asked you at the beginning where you wanted it.'

He doesn't hear. He's as angry as those steel hammers. He couldn't risk letting go until now.

'We never should have left when we did, we weren't ready.' He stares at me like I'm to blame. 'If you weren't so determined to get away, we could have prepared properly. The problems we had weren't necessary.'

He doesn't get angry. The sea has turned him inside out. I won't take him too seriously, he's old. I don't want to cry inside.

'We should've taken Jack and Emily sailing first.' He jumps around. 'If you hadn't been so set on leaving early, Jack would have known how scared he was and he wouldn't have come. He shouldn't have come.'

Jack nods, he can't help it.

I whine back. There's not a lot of power in my words either.

'Dad, you said you don't have shake-down cruises anymore because you always lose your crew.'

He turns away – he's not a saint.

'There's far too much mess everywhere. It's impossible to sail a boat safely in this state.'

I stop. The trip was too hard. I don't feel guilty because I couldn't do any more. He's mainly worried about his computer. It's been days on its side in a puddle of stale beer.

'Okay, let's have some music. Emily, you help me clean up.'

Hot water bubbles on the stove. Eva Cassidy's melodious voice wafts through the boat. We make big piles of washing and big piles of rubbish. I shake the woolly white rugs and lay them smoothly on the bunks. I sweep and scrub. Jack goes into the cockpit to hunt for cups and empty beer cans. He wipes the crumbs and collects the scraps, pieces of chocolate and ragged bags of nuts. Emily fills the sink with hot bubbly water for the dishes. I put the books and charts away. We each tend our festering tiredness and disappointment alone, until the boat is finally shipshape.

Jack is fishing with a piece of rotting salami.

'Hey, Jack,' I peek up. 'Do you think you'll catch a fish for our dinner?'

'Nup.'

Emily shrinks behind her book. She could feel guilty, but stays gloomy and angry instead. Dad rests.

'Anyone for a cup of tea?'

'Thanks, Alice. I'll have one with you,' he smiles.

The big clean-up helped. It's the only time we worked as a team, the whole trip. 'Dad, tell us some more about Fiji?'

'Well, from what I've heard Fijian culture was about as barbaric as you get. Old people like me were strangled; the sick were buried alive; the odd shipwrecked sailor was mercilessly cooked and eaten.'

I climb out on deck to scan the new city. We can't go ashore until tomorrow when customs and quarantine clear us. I sit in the cockpit to brood on that great creature carrying us. Life evolved in the sea. The sea runs in my veins. The sea held us on her back for fourteen days. I am embedded in the sea.

Emily curtly asks where my tent is. Jack hovers in the background, counting down the seconds. Dad gruffly steps around their packs to go outside and check the weather.

Freedom is a superficial inspection away and quarantine and customs officials arrive early. The smiling dark-skinned natives inspect our passports, hand us some forms to fill in and welcome us to Fiji. Jack can hardly contain his excitement. I drag the crumpled dinghy from the front berth and pump it up. We toss it overboard. Dad produces a brand new two-stroke outboard.

'I'll make the mixture a little richer for its maiden voyage, so the pistons wear in gently.' He pours oil generously into the petrol. The motor starts easily and we push off.

'What's wrong?' we collectively call as the motor splutters into silence. Dad whips it into action a couple more times, but it then falls into an unshakeable groaning. The fresh wind blowing out of the harbour catches the broad side of our dinghy and takes off with us.

'Grab the side of that big Russian fishing boat,' Dad shouts. We act quickly. 'Good,' he says. 'We can pull ourselves under its bowsprit and around to the ladder.' This is almost fun. 'Alice, go see if someone has a screwdriver.'

I climb the ladder. Three Russian sailors appear and they don't speak English, but they do understand my request, 'A spanner?'

Dad stays calm, like he's been in this kind of situation before. I'm sure he has been! Jack, the helicopter pilot with exceptionally high standards of technical competence, fumes. The engine starts, wind blows the dinghy, and Emily in particular, under a waterfall pumping from the fishing boat's bilge. We wave our relief to the crew, but it is short-lived. Jack and I row to the wharf.

Jack would explode into a thousand pieces of rage if I poked him. As soon as our passports are stamped, he and Emily leave, bouncing packs along the coconut palms to pursue their freedom. Dad and I row to the yacht club for lunch and cold beer. The outboard can wait.

I want to walk into town. Dad would take a taxi. We need the exercise. Slapping our jandals we cross the tarseal and concrete, striding past untidy businesses, stepping in front of cars, exhaust fumes and dust blowing us around. Coconut palms alone wave our tropical dream. Dad trots with short sharp steps, to keep up. Being on land is a shock. The deep ocean is no longer swelling through us, rolling us unsteadily steady, in unending movement. But the land has fresh vegetables and fruit – pawpaws, watermelons, small fist-shaped tomatoes and long thin-legged eggplants – down at the market. The fruit is sweet and brightly-coloured. Big, proud, good-looking people with broad grins and lots of children move around us. Fiji is our new adventure. I become desperate to dive into this anonymous mass of brown humanity – this is why I sailed away.

Smiling young men come to our rescue back at the yacht club. It seems the mixture in the fuel tank is too rich. I paddle my feet in the tide on a concrete breakwater while they empty the tank, carefully measure the correct proportions of oil and petrol, and refill it. We motor confidently back out to *Dream-maker*, into an empty space, for a fresh start.

I start reading *The Totorore Voyage*, about a fellow kiwi on a three-and-a-half-year sailing voyage around Chile and Antarctica, studying the population distribution of birds.

'Dad, we weren't the only ones with problems. Gerry Clark set out without shake-down cruises.'

I read out how his crew lay seasick for weeks, leaving him to cook and sail the boat alone. He sailed into endless gale-force winds a couple of days out, like we did. His battery wouldn't hold a charge no matter what he did. He had bilge pump problems, wind vane problems, wind generator problems, leaks and more. Dad and I smile.

'Problems are normal,' I reassure him.

Dad smiles weakly. He's made this trip before.

'Someone's boarding,' he says.

'Hi, Mum, it's just us. We need a few more clothes.' Their dinghy ride putters away.

'I can't take you back in right now,' Dad snaps. 'The outboard's still playing up. I need to empty it again.'

Jack knew it was a mistake to come back. He grabs a handful of beers and retreats to the cockpit. He won't come down, he won't talk, he won't eat. He drinks, calming himself into an alcoholic haze.

Dad fills up with wine and whiskey and puts on the 'Seekers'.

I turn to Emily. 'I sang these songs to you as a baby. I haven't heard them in twenty years.'

'You know, Alice, I've been alone on my yacht so many times, unloved and abandoned by life, but I've always pulled through.' Dad's voice is a little slurred.

Emily curls in the corner, intrigued, wishing she was somewhere else, grumpy and not knowing why.

'Dad, you're an adventurer. Adventurers have to face loneliness – it's part of their story.'

When 'Strauss Waltzes' come on, he jumps up from his seat, red nosed and effusive, a resurrected Dean Martin, dancing with a woman in his arms.

'I have enjoyed so many women in my time. They've all been good to me.'

Next morning I stay while Dad takes Emily and Jack ashore. One of my straggly branches has got caught up in Dad's and I can't shake myself free. I seem to have climbed my way over into his tree. He has a lot to say about Jack and Emily. I don't even want to think about them. I want to get on with my life.

'Emily and Jack both need to grow up. They shouldn't have come back after they'd left. It wasn't right for them to leave the way they did, when we were having trouble with the outboard motor.'

I don't care. Does he think I agree when I don't say anything? I stomp around now he's not here, festering. I stare back into his eyes of resentment and disappointment. When he's here, I daren't meet his gaze.

On his return, I make a salad lunch and we sit down with a bottle of wine.

'Young people have gone soft on it. Now, in my day I was running a whole post office by the time I was sixteen. I went to war at seventeen.'

'I know, Dad. Life is a lot more complicated now.' I try to be objective, but I get caught in his branches every time.

'Life didn't begin for me until I was in my fifties,' he starts again. 'The 1960s and '70s were the time of encounter groups. Encounter groups changed my life. I realised my life belonged to me and it was up to me to make the life I wanted. I didn't belong to other people.' He pauses for another gulp of wine. 'From then on I dreamed of nothing but freedom, day and night. I couldn't get the word out of my head. Finally, I sailed away. I sailed away.' He almost looks at me. 'I woke up to the great adventure living can be. The world is your oyster and it's Emily's too. You can do anything you want.'

I pour another glass of wine while he launches off again.

'We create our own lives, you know. The world is what we think it is. You can have any reality you want.'

My hackles start to rise. Such grandiose delusion annoys the hell out of me. He's totally forgotten our earlier conversation.

'But Dad, of course that's not true.'

I stop. What's the point? He just pruned all my branches to bare stumps.

He continues: 'We are what we think we are. The limitation is in your mind, not reality. Reality is limitless. We grow and die old because we think we will. Change the thought and reality must change.'

I want to scream. We've had this conversation too many times – it takes too much energy to bring it to life, to think of something new to say, to be creative and fresh.

'Dad, we both know that you can't possibly think your way out of dying.'

I know what he is trying to say, but he's all confused. I agree that the 'word' came first, but it was the word of God, not man.

Dad has a ready reply. 'I'm divine, a God within. As the mind of God, I'm responsible for everything I have ever done or experienced. I created my whole life.'

I want to throw something at him. How can he talk like this – he doesn't have any idea what he is talking about. It's all talk, and it's talk about what is so precious to me.

'We create a life of limitation by accepting limiting beliefs. Life is limitless.'

'But Dad, there's no such thing as unlimited thought, it's a contradiction in terms. Can't you see that once a choice is made, which it must be, the world becomes limited.'

He doesn't hear me. 'When you realise that you are God then you will have power over life and death.'

He stops in the force of his pronouncement, even though all his experience says the opposite. How can I take this conversation seriously? He is getting old and will certainly die soon.

'Dad, of course you are going to die and so am I. We need to rest.'

There is a lot to admire in my father, but at times he frustrates the hell out of me.

This is our life on an ocean wave – the flotsam and jetsam of ideas thrashing uselessly around the lunch table, neither dissolving back into the unmade source, nor transforming into a thing of beauty. These ideas appear again and again at every turning tide. I want to gather them up and make a great fire so we can begin again. I grab the Buddha's teaching as a lifeline. The enlightened being has no fixed views or opinions. No enlightened being ensnares life with his words, crucifying the living on the cross of a fixed view or considered position, clinging to beliefs over the dead bodies of those he has passed judgement on. The Buddha mind is rooted in the endlessly changing, empty ocean.

7

The heat is unpleasant; the tiny breeze flickering through the open hatch is teasingly inadequate. It rains. Each day a few more yachts thread their way into the quiet waters of the harbour. Rubber dinghies motor or row between shore and boat. Rusting hulls of large fishing boats snuggle together in twos and threes. An occasional boat minder wanders the deck to take some air. Night approaches. I stomp back and forth in my prison. I need to walk. Suddenly I remember my dream of the ocean. It arrives to wake me up, to remind me that I am not my unsteady thoughts. I may be disgruntled, but this isn't me. I'm as still and free as the deep steady ocean beneath the churning waves. 'Being disgruntled' is free to stay or go; it doesn't matter to me. I dive and surface, back and forth, waves and ocean.

'Dad, let's go ashore.'

We motor in with bags of rubbish and an empty water container and happen to bump into a young American couple we met at customs. They were leaving but it's raining and they come in with us for a drink. Liz is bubbly and talkative; her young husband falls into his chair like a sleepy bear. They're sailing indefinitely until the money runs out. She and I arrange to catch up in the morning at large concrete washing tubs around the back of the yacht club.

I row back out to *Dream-maker* in the drizzling dark, the outboard a defeated shadow behind Dad.

He breaks the silence. 'I think we should stay in Fiji and forget about Vanuatu and Noumea.' We wobble past the first boat. 'Fiji's a beautiful place. Sailing home from Noumea is difficult, but from Fiji we should have a good cross wind all the way.'

Marion, my sister, warned me. She said he wouldn't want to move.

'Dad, that's not what you promised. We have six months. I couldn't stand being stuck in this harbour for six months.'

'Why are you so restless?' A dull light hits the side of his face. 'There is so much to explore here. You haven't seen anything yet.'

The oars whip up sheets of spray, slapping and biting the water. Lumpy muscle bulges through my loose shirt. 'That's not fair. It's not what we agreed to. We missed Tonga and Samoa and now you want to stay here. I want to see the world, not just Fiji.'

I have no sympathy with his tiredness; I have no sympathy for my own. I need to grab myself and remember I'm not this angry person, I'm not the froth on the sea, stirred this way and that by every passing wind. I rush for the safety of the dark warm ocean. This argument with Dad isn't real.

Doing nothing in calm waters, I become out of sorts and wrestle free from my sarong and squirm under simple love songs playing on the radio. A hollow sense that life is about being young and in love sinks me. Where are all the people I love? I grab Dad's computer and write emails onto a CD. I scribble postcards to send home. I miss everyone. I want to be appreciated. Dad waits for me to finish, sipping his second coffee. I grab my journal; I don't want to be his daughter.

Suva is a jumble of containers for selling things: facades of glass and aluminium, colonially-turned balustrades, peeling paintwork, large concrete boxes. Like my deformed tree, branching out from a rootless trunk, it doesn't hold together in a beautiful way. Yesterday, sitting in the scrap of a park, I watched the pedestrians coming and going, striding long, swelling like the sea, ebbing and flowing along the pavement. They live through their bodies. Back home, we jerk our bodies along with our heads, disconnected. I swallow grape-seed oil, CoQ10, royal jelly, yeast, Panadol, B vitamins – anything I can find tossing around on the boat to fix me.

Dad's reprimanding me, in my head, like a cracked record: 'Life is for living. The world is a wonderful place. Your theories about suffering are so negative. I don't believe in suffering. My life has been full of happiness. I have had a wonderful life. Why can't you relax?' His face is torn between concern and annoyance. Where the hell does all of that leave me? I can't be who he wants me to be. I want to crawl into a hole and die.

Dad runs the noisy, smelly generator. He makes tea around the mess and clutter of tools and clothes and rags. I start tidying up so he doesn't see how I am. Projects are on the go all around us. He's taken up the floorboards so he can get at the bilge. He's planted the batteries in the middle of the table. The outboard motor is in pieces on the two main bunks. I can't stand it. In meditation, we train ourselves to sit through uncomfortable feelings, to stay present – without moving, without doing anything – looking calmly into whatever arises until the distress unravels, until it changes its face. If I can stay here, maybe I will discover something, but I am far too uncomfortable to stay. I want to be off, 'not moving', somewhere else.

I stomp around on deck in the fresh air, as far away from Dad as possible. It seems to me that as soon as I get beneath the exciting stories to tell back home – the romance of a tropical paradise – as soon as I get down to the nitty-gritty of my ordinary day, a lot of it's pretty awful. What would Dad find if he looked honestly into his actual feelings, his thoughts? I bet he would find a solid landfill of suffering: a shadow land of discomfort, disappointment and resentment. Is this why we all spend so much time drifting away in our minds? We can't stand to be anywhere near here.

Jack arrives to collect his things – fiery orange hair, keen face, strong lean body all pointing to everything we're not. The need to pick up his clothes destroyed his resolve to never set foot on a boat ever again. He and Emily have been fighting and they've been sick.

'I'm not sure what Emily's thinking about us at the moment. She seems pretty unhappy.'

'That must be hard for you,' I sympathise. 'I can't imagine a more testing time than the one you've had. Maybe it'll turn out okay in the end?'

'I hope so. I'm looking forward to getting home.'

He stays, but not long enough for a cup of tea.

He has an airplane ticket, so we can sign him off at customs. He and Emily have another week before he leaves. Then she'll come back to the boat. I'm not holding my breath.

I visit the museum in the afternoon. The Fijians originally came from Southeast Asia, four thousand years ago. A further migration of Melanesians from Southeast Asia arrived one thousand seven hundred years ago. I peer inside the glass cases. The intricate style of early pottery devolves into functional, unornamented kitchen bowls. The houses and boats in the middle of the room lack any decoration or fine detail. I move slowly from one display to the next. Groups of uniformed school children come and go, and the odd visitor. Religious beliefs seem poorly developed – they aren't even mentioned. Unritualised cannibalism was widespread. Female infanticide was common and young boys were given enemy children to practice killing.

In a new room, I peer down into a glass case full of intricate carvings and fine brocades, precious jewellery and beautiful saris. The gods are well and truly alive here. Brahma and Shiva subdued and refined the Indian mind in a beautiful way. Indians are small and slender – they use their minds to survive. Fijians are big and strong. Only the very strong made it through the coral traps of the Pacific and the treacherous reefs around Fiji.

What a difference! I suddenly realise that culture is the enduring, evolving shape of humanity. I never shaped my life, I was never in charge. I am the product of my culture. I grew up through its schools and TV programmes; I wear its thoughts and behaviour. Culture is the organism. I'm an experimental cell. Sobering. I will forget – I will think myself centre stage again, the creator of my life, just the way Dad says.

I walk through unkempt botanical gardens, a reminder of Fiji's colonial past. A young Fijian crosses my path. We chat, his eyes imploring. 'Please marry me,' he pleads.

I laugh him off in a friendly way. He stands in my way, submissive yet demanding. 'Let me look into your eyes? Please take your glasses off.'

'You've got to be kidding.'

How did he get to thinking this would work? He is attractive in a soft way.

'What's your name?' he asks.

I remain elusive, impassively cool behind my sunglasses. I keep walking until I bump into another local along the waterfront, the rare half Indian-half Fijian. He's fishing.

'Hello.' I slow down to see if he's caught anything.

He returns my greeting. 'Do you know anything about that group of people over there?' He points to an assortment of locals and white people.

'No.' We chat. He stands and talks like someone who is comfortable in his life, in a good way. I'm always curious about this possibility. I'm relieved the Fijians have been civilised by the white man – it means I'm safe. The villages are relatively peaceful. Battered old buses and orange cordial stands rub shoulders with Pajero's and cappuccino cafés. Strong young men in their twenties and thirties sell glasses of iced juice down at the bus station.

The harbour bounces in the wind. I check my washing a couple of times through the night. Safety-pinned or threaded through the line, it should be fine. The undies look playful, but not about to make a great leap for freedom. I need to make a leap for freedom. Jaded and grumpy, I go back ashore to the park. Under another tree, I'm approached almost immediately by another young man, as a potential ticket out of here. We chat and start out for an internet café before I get it. What on earth was I thinking?

'I'm sorry. I don't want to be doing this.'

I leave him looking nonplussed and head in the opposite direction to buy lunch from a café on the main street.

'Are you sure you want to eat inside?' the Chinese owner asks persistently.

'Sure. I need to sit down to eat.' I sit alone at a small table as a dozen youngsters, girls and boys, laugh and smoke and pass around large bottles of Fijian beer next to me.

At an email café, I check my mail. James and I went out for a bit and became friends, with a kind of 'maybe when we're old and desperately single' understanding. Happy to hear from him, I fall into a cloud of romantic fantasy. He sounds depressed – another failed romance, I expect. We sailed his yacht a few times, or rather he sailed and I looked pretty holding the tiller. I happily send off some more letters to my children and friends.

Stuck in Suva until Emily arrives, I spend hours sitting out on deck, away from the clutter of Dad's thoughts and projects. Sometimes the wind and sea feed me, sometimes my thoughts feed me.

The proud carriage of the Fijians fascinates me. I want to know about the kind of tree they are, rooted solidly in the ground. I keep losing myself in my spindly branches, then I have to go away to find my roots again, and then I'm not even sure what it is I've found. I sit with these images, the differences, and suddenly jump up with excitement. That's it – the secret of eternal youth. To stay forever young is to stay forever given up to life. Youth is all about life bubbling through. Age is all about stagnant dead ends.

A lone grey heron feeds at the breakwater. I pass it often when I'm rowing. I'd wondered whether it was lonely, its small grey-feathered body so separate from the gracefully-falling palm fronds and rocky breakwater. Now I can see that it lives the glancing golden light and the ocean slapping at its feet.

I like being out in the breeze, where my mind is free to wonder. Where does Dad's mind go to escape feeling lonely? Does he wrestle metaphysical perspectives, or is he full of the fuss and bother of boat stuff? Does he wander into fantasy to make the day okay, or does his mind go blank? Mine does all these things.

The wind blows in, so I'm always looking into port, away from the misty green hills. Sea-battered fishing boats from all over the world tie up together at the wharves. Hanging low above the water, some are more rust than paint. They are being repaired and refitted so they can return to sea. A young couple with three children wave as they pass and then I'm stranded again with these old fishing boats.

Dad pokes his head up. 'Alice, I want to move the boat further out. If a westerly blows, we'll end up onshore here.'

I follow him down into the smoky saloon, tuna-tin ashtray full of stubs. I don't want to move.

'Look.' I point to the barometer. 'A westerly only blows if a storm is coming. If a storm was coming the barometer would be falling. Isn't that what you told me?'

'I don't care, I want to move.'

I raise the anchor and Dad edges us around. The sea goes red.

'We're aground. I'll have to reverse,' is his answer to my worried look.

Stuck in mud, that's us. We run aground a second time. Further than I can now row ashore, I drop anchor. There are at least twenty boats swinging between us and the shore.

A Japanese couple motor over almost immediately. The young woman springs up to grab our boat; her companion, an old toothless man huddles in the back.

'The anchorage here is no good because the mud's too soft. We dragged a couple of nights ago and ended up tangled in those fishing boats. An American couple also dragged, so be careful.'

She restarts their motor, smiles and zooms off.

Nowhere is safe for us now.

'The wind's coming up. We'll put down a second anchor,' Dad frets. 'You'll find the second anchor and some chain in the lazaret. You need to shackle them together.'

I move oily rags and a wrench and a container of screws to make a space to cook in. I'll go camping for a few days! Dad can concentrate on his projects. Parked on the navigation table is a new belt for the alternator; the bilge pump has moved to the cockpit for daylight inspection; floor boards are leaning against the beds; the mouldy fridge is getting mouldier; the outboard is back together and ready for another trial run; and our new batteries are on shore being properly recharged. I glue broken wings back on the wind charger.

8

Laden with my pack and tent I plonk myself down on a broken bus seat. The bus rattles out of town and through the outlying villages – rusting corrugated iron houses painted dirty pinks and yellows, swept earth yards with chickens, dogs and children running free under large breadfruit and mango trees. A few plastered and tiled posh houses hide behind locked iron gates. I'm on my way to a tourist hideaway next to Colo-i-Suva, the national forest park. The bus drops me on a winding road, wild jungle all around, overcast sky above, my destination around the next bend – I hope.

'Yes, you can pitch a tent by the lake. It does rain a lot and it gets cold at night. Enjoy your stay.'

The small lake is a greeny-brown soup of mud and algae. I unclip my tent and shake it out. Where are they? I search the folds and underneath – no tent pegs. I will never lend my tent to my children again. I won't let it matter. Twigs will hold well enough if it doesn't blow or rain too much. I erect the tent efficiently and professionally in case someone is watching. I'm sure no one is. The whole front unzips onto the water view and I sink into the soft ground – into all the times and places I've been alone in my tent – giggling because there's nowhere else to go, no further to fall. I'm safe. Blue is gone. I'm surrounded by a myriad yellow-green floating, swaying, sighing leaves.

Across the grass volleyball court is the shower – warm if I'm lucky. It's cold. I walk onto the grey-metalled road. Birds sip nectar way above me, hopping across blossoms and singing. I stroll through grey drizzle to the entrance of the forest park, vacant inside, a hint of nothing moving, and back home through the same grey drizzle, nudging forlorn, then up the long driveway, right across the volleyball court back to my tent, then across to the kitchen with an onion, a tin of tuna and some rice, mechanical mind.

Focused on the onion under the sharp blade of my Swiss army knife, I start a simple dinner, sharing the kitchen with a couple of young backpackers. There are so many names for people like us: tourist, backpacker, traveller, visitor, holidaymaker, wanderer and hobo – a different name for a different purpose. I pick 'wanderer', because I'm unsure where I'm heading in the short term. We chat, sharing stories in the setting sun and I write down the name of a possible destination, Na-nui-ra.

Now I can meditate. Crosslegged in my tent on my Thermarest chair, I lean back to take the pressure off my knees and settle my mind into the spreading space. I bring awareness to my body, to the sensations: heavy, dull, clear, soft. This expands the sensation and takes my mind inside. The sensations keep changing, almost dancing. I note textures, associated feelings and memories. My mind deepens, inner voices chatter softly in the background as I settle into my belly, round and full. The candle lantern swings on its knot to keep the night at bay. In the background a saintly choir from the local church sounds through my body.

Suddenly I am distracted by the thought of food and a cup of coffee. Mindfulness slip into mindlessness and, without even thinking, I follow my impulse back into the night and kitchen and bathroom where giggling girls struggle with a cold shower that turns hot in bursts, and their shrieking fingers point to a giant spider hiding in the shower curtain.

Morning is overcast and still. Shimmering palm fronds, clumps of taro and delicate tree ferns rise from the mirrored surface of the cloudy lake. Girls preen themselves in front of large mirrors, roosters crow their self-importance. I hug my tea on a bench seat by the lake, fret about my children, and fall into the confused stories I left behind in New Zealand. Now rain-coated, with snacks in the pocket, I start out through drizzling rain to the forest park.

'Do you want a guide?' they ask at the entrance.

'No, thank you. I'll be fine on my own. I'll stay on the path.'

They send someone to watch over me all the same. I have been a long time away from the bush, the silent, majestic trees. A shadowy keeper follows in the background.

The bush is my place of pilgrimage. For years I tramped the national parks of New Zealand, dragging and enticing my children, cajoling friends. We'd stagger from the dripping bush and collapse in the golden tussock. I spent weeks roaming the high country alone, tripping along the lace of powdery snow.

I walk on, past large water holes. Is it safe to swim alone? Is it too cold? I stop thinking and dive right in.

Dusk arrives as I return home, a simple wanderer, dirty and wet. Last night was cold so I plump up with all the clothes in my pack. The candle lantern swings wildly.

In the morning I peel off the outer layers, remake my Thermarest seat, reorganise my bags and bits and pieces to tidy up and start meditating again. I didn't bring much food; I get tired of thinking about food but I still get hungry. Ants found the snap-lock bag of nuts and raisins in the night, so now I only have porridge for breakfast, two oranges for lunch, rice and a few vegetables for dinner. I gave away my second tin of tuna.

My mind – I'm always noticing how my mind is – grows cool and steady. Distracting thoughts fade before turning into the hooks they might become. I get ready for my walk. My mind is spacious and clear. Laughter hangs in the air around me, going nowhere. The chattering of workmen is pure melody, no reaction. The long-nosed kingfisher close by watches from its dead tree-limb.

Although the day is clear and warm, yesterday's rain still hangs in the trees. My mind slips in ahead of me, into the leaves and branches fanning out wide. White water falls over black rock, inside the cascading, tumbling water. A trail of broken rock, rock consciousness, slipping into silent rock pools and large boulders. I follow the steps carved in slippery rock. Dark hardwood planks carry me over side streams tumbling into the bush while cool plants caress me back to my body. By another rock pool, I rest under the dark eaves of a thatched picnic table. Misty half-thoughts float by, like the mist of yesterday's rain. Luxuriant plants coax the light, bursting with triumph, 'We are alive.' I dive into a pool again and roll around swimming.

Sun warms my shamelessly bare limbs as I stroll the wide gravel road home. Everything is flowing, I am flowing. I skirt big puddles of thick red clay while the breeze plays with my hair and sarong. The road and I are crossing like ribbons, meeting and re-meeting. I dart off along a side track down to more pools. Yesterday there were children and families swimming; today I'm mostly alone.

On the long walk home a police car stops. Two softly-spoken uniformed Fijians question me: 'Are you all right? Where have you come from? Where are you going?'

I hear later that a white woman was raped here a year ago.

The night becomes dark quite suddenly, starless and moonless. My torchlight flickers over the lake and back, to find a path across the stones and grass volley-ball court. The dim light shines on wet leaf litter. There, at the far side of the resort, a shadow, my tent, sagging under all the rain that fell.

In a tent not far from mine, a young English backpacker starts screaming at her boyfriend. In the dark, up on the hill, a Fijian woman shouts recklessly at her man. I recognize the pain, the need to rail against a man. I cringe and snuggle down into my bed to remember the tranquil Zen garden and soothing clear water.

Morning arrives. Snuggled in my sleeping bag, my eyes reluctantly open. The tent is a radiant emerald-green, a stunning, light-enhanced extravagance. Once before, my sense of smell exploded and I found myself building a fine three-dimensional smell picture of my world, tracing the passage of a smell as it wove around other smells, sensing where a smell had come from and where it was going. Now, my seeing has burst open another dimension of light. I fold up the tent, pack my bag and stroll through the resort. I'm ready to go. I sit at the bar table and then perch on a porcelain toilet, noticing a layer of significance swimming around me. I made it here, into this world. I'm part of an endless stream of people who have leaned on this table and sat on this toilet. I am the mind of man, triumphant, like the plants in the forest. Nothing more is required. I throw my pack up onto my back, now jubilant, and return to the open road.

The morning bus returns me the way I came, winding down the outer settlements of Suva into the dusty clutter of the market place. Dad is expecting me sometime today – evening if I like. Clutching an iced juice, roti and steam cake I find shade on the edge of a wooden crate. I like the way the earth has turned itself into food, painting itself into bright colours and funny shapes, piled high into pyramids of oranges, clumping up into knuckle-bone tomatoes, squashed purple kumara, and long, long beans spilling onto the ground. Cabbages, lettuces, spring onions and carrots, an endless variety spread out over the long tables. Large wands of aromatic kava and paper bags of its fine powder musk the air. Indians weigh rice and pungent spices into clear cellophane packets. Outside, women and children eat in the shade, and guard their wares spreading out on the ground.

I decide to go for a two-and-a-half-hour bus ride to Pacific Harbour, a tourist destination up the coast, and fumble for change in my waist pouch. With my pack slung over one shoulder, free hand clutching paper bag snacks, water bottle about to fall from its high perch, I move myself down the bus aisle to an empty seat. As I crash into the seat, the water bottle tumbles and rolls underneath. I look down into the market and imagine the lives of the women and their men. Are they are happy? Through the window, I buy peanuts from a young boy. Am I happy? A spiritual teacher once told me that all we're looking for is happiness. I love long bus rides – this time for contemplation.

The bus follows flat land along the coast. It rumbles past Indian settlements – neatly laid-out houses with grubby plastered, arched verandahs – and clatters past Fijian villages where broken fibrolite and rusting corrugated iron cling to rotting wood in a more communal way. Derelict shacks peep from a wasteland of scrub and grass. Endless strings of washing dry in the wind.

'Domestic violence is a big problem among the Fijians. We go into the villages to teach the men. They won't accept the government law telling them not to abuse their women.' Police officials told me this at the forest park.

'Virtually all Indian marriages are arranged. The suicide rate is very high among the Indians,' an aid worker told me at the backpackers.

The day is grey and bleak. I wonder about the lives of these people. It seems, from the bus window, they must be pretty grey and bleak as well. If they stopped to look at their lives – the hardship, the distractions they cultivate so they don't have to look – what then?

The bus keeps rumbling along, past yet more untidy settlements. I imagine arguments – establishing power, fighting over money, lies, status.

I carry a plate of food and coffee to my table under a covered verandah at Pacific Harbour. Rain pours down solidly. Pop music and voices merge with its sullen despairing tone. I sit in the rain and reflect on my situation. I pick at my cake and reject an offer by the hairdresser to cut my hair. It's long and wild – I don't want it tamed. I order another cup of coffee.

I think back to what I learned on my cycling trip. As a young child, I fell from grace through the jaws of time. I solidified out as a creature of flesh and blood, caught running after pleasure and away from pain. My human mind turned love into desire and fear, and awareness into thought. This is what happened to me. I became reduced to a marionette in life's dance. I trotted off to kindergarten in gingham and frills and to school in pinafores and long white socks. I was very protective of a sense of 'self' ballooning through my consciousness. By the time I had adopted the navy gym tunic and stockings of high school, the mind mirrors reflecting me to myself were solid walls. I was angry all the time, but I didn't know it.

And then one day, when I was thirty-two, a hand reached down. A friend led me to the house of a spiritual teacher. For the first time, I realized I didn't work properly. I needed to change, but in order to change I needed to find out how I had been made. The tide was turning. With the objective rigour of a scientist, I started to look at the mess inside me. I teased apart my behaviour, emotions, motives, guilt, fear, problems with trust, my relationship to my mother.

My second coffee cup is empty. It's still raining. The passionate courage I found in my thirties starts beating all over again. Life will never again be that magnificent breaststroke through the shimmering border between what I knew and what I didn't know about myself and life. Meditation was the best adventure I had ever been on. I shake free of my contemplations and look for a distraction. Window shopping will do. The nearest souvenir shop is full of carved four-pronged wooden forks – big ones, small ones, some implanted with shell, some bound in plaited string – used in primitive times to pick at deliciously-roasted human brain. Now they carve them for tourists. Behind the shops is a thatched walkway and stage for entertaining tourists. I walk into the garden, around the showers of rain. I realize that self awareness is a precious flower of the human mind.

M any years ago I became fascinated with exploring the consciousness inside other life forms. I tunnelled into dark interior space, way down inside my body, on a slender thread of awareness, without any adornment. I never knew where I was going in those days, I just waited to see. One day, in the scary amorphous dark interior of myself, beyond myself, this slender thread spontaneously grew into the dim consciousness of a cell, as a myriad sensations of movement, flickering light and dark, moving towards, moving away from, tasting. As a cell I was having a primitive mental experience, at least that's how I understood my experience. Mind and matter were two fundamental aspects of all life.

I kept going. Another time, from the dark interior– dim as a tiny torch going out – my consciousness shaped itself into the mind of a cat, crystal clear and sharply focused. The mind shocked me. I couldn't stop to think whether I wanted to hunt or not – I had to hunt. I was barely self-conscious, but keenly present. The cat had no way out of its situation, its actions were determined. My human mind was different. I still didn't understand what this mind was for, where it was headed, but it was magnificent.

The rain is over and so am I. I shake raindrops from my hair, put away my journal and stroll over to catch the last bus of the day. An eager taxi driver offers a fare so close to the bus fare I can't refuse and I return in upholstered comfort to the busy metropolis of Suva.

9

Emily sees Jack off at the airport and returns to the boat. We are leaving the same day with a few hours to wash clothes, buy food, buy wire for new tent pegs, check emails, refuel and re-water. I dally over my emails.

'Come on, we still have to put the water in the tanks.' Emily prods.

She folds her things away neatly in our tidy boat. Dad motors us out past the old fishing boats, away from the cacophonous wharf. I pull up the main with delight, and follow its flapping all the way up the mast. Two weeks at anchor was quite long enough for the headsail; it leaps out jubilantly to catch the wind. Dad turns *Dream-maker* away from the wind until the breeze is straight across the beam, then I take the helm while he sets the wind vane.

'Now I'll show you both something of Fiji. You'll see how beautiful the islands are.' He beams, alive in his memories.

'Mum, I'm worried about being seasick again.'

'You'll be okay. We aren't going far. You can be in charge of the meals while we're sailing, okay?'

She nods, matching my confidence, and disappears into the galley to make tea, open a packet of biscuits and find a smile. She can do it. I watch her peel cucumber and carrots for a salad, tossing her head back self-consciously, dismissing my concern.

Beqa, a solitary small bush-covered isle, rises over the horizon and floats out of the sea towards us. Dad noses into its sheltered bay, eye on the depth finder.

'Alice, drop the anchor here,' he calls.

I stand on the rubber mount to start the windlass. The anchor chain rattles out of the hawsepipe and carries the anchor down through liquid crystal into golden sand. *Dream-maker* swings around into the wind and golden tussock-covered slopes and dark forested valleys swing into view. Emily gazes ashore to the long empty beach lined with coconut palms. This is her dream of Fiji. It's mine as well. I want to kick my feet through the sand, pant up the hills brushing windswept hair from my face and fall into the long grass on the summit.

Late afternoon light is still tunnelling through the water so, snorkelled up, we all fall off the boat to explore the shimmering underwater kingdom of darting fish and coral gardens – our first time snorkelling in Fiji. Dappled light bounces off the quivering, multi-coloured fish poking their way around extravagant forests of coral. I'm on the outside of their lives. The fish move differently from creatures on land; they hover in tentative groups and slip past hesitantly. Corals are colonies of coelenterates, primitive sea-anemone animals growing bold colourful shapes with hard and brittle limbs. We don't recognise each other.

Emily dives and flippers around energetically. She's finally getting into her holiday. She can tell her friends about snorkelling. Dad goes through the motions of swimming.

We haul ourselves back onto the boat as the sun dies. Soaking up our dream, coconut palms in the background, I cook up sausages with kumara and cabbage and pass the loaded plates into the cockpit.

'Dad, here's a warm beer. This place is beautiful. I can't wait to go ashore tomorrow.'

He answers abruptly: 'I want to leave early in the morning. You won't be able to go ashore. This is not a secure anchorage. If the wind turns we'll be on a lee shore.'

The catch is that nowhere outside a harbour is safe, but harbours are boring. I sit alone on deck and follow shadowy waves back to the mountains of mainland Fiji in the distance, back into the great brooding creature called life. Surely my destiny, the destiny of humankind upon this planet, is to know ourselves in the richest possible way, to bring into our knowing this great brooding nurturing planet, which over millions of years wove us into being. We are inextricably each other.

I wake several times in the night from difficult dreams. However, I'm not lost in the sweeping, crashing anxiety – I'm the unshakeable calm of the ocean, the container of the stories. This is progress.

I drift into the smell of Indian spices, nuts and raisins boiling on the stove.

'Mum, are you awake? I've made tea and porridge.' The old Emily is back.

My eyes open softly. I can see by the way she's moving she's happy. The whole of her is stirring the porridge. The quizzical look on her face says, 'Why isn't life always so simple and satisfying?' She's bathed in glassy, rippled, emerald light.

'How peculiar. It's like we're still in the sea and you're a colourful, translucent fish. Everything is luminous, with golden light pouring out.'

She smiles. 'Here's your tea, Mum.'

'Alice, we're leaving this morning. It's time to wake up.' Dad's making sure I'm not going to drift away somewhere else.

'Okay, okay.' I look outside. There's almost no wind. 'Are you sure you want to go today?'

'Yes, this is not a secure anchorage.'

I empty my porridge bowl and spring up on deck. Full of nuts and raisins, I'm ready to go.

'Dad, I'm ready with the anchor.'

'I didn't mean we had to leave right now.' He follows me out and starts the engine, still chewing his toast.

The main goes up easily in the light wind. Most times it gets caught around something. Usually the reefing lines curl back on themselves and lock against the hole they're meant to be running back into, or a lazy jack catches the edge of the sail and locks it fast, or a reefing line catches around something on deck. There are endless variations to my call, 'Dad, the sail's stuck!'

Today it goes up smoothly, without a hitch, almost all the way by hand. I'm strong now and winch only for the stretch. Smiling into the cockpit, I let the headsail out – actually it pretty much blows itself out – and winch it in to Dad's instructions. Emily's washed the dishes and tidied the galley. Now she's sunbathing topless on the upside-down rubber dinghy at the front of the boat.

I have boxfuls of photos at home of me and my sisters sunbathing on deck. Sailing for us as teenagers was about getting the blackest tan possible and taking the wheel when required.

'Can I join you for an overall tan as well?' I ask.

Yesterday we had fun getting ready to snorkel as we sorted through a jumble of bikini bits from second-hand shops, looking for matching pieces. We disappeared into the tumbling chaos that poured out of the wardrobe, our differences humbled by the endless quantities of stuff. I had packed so many possible adventures in there on top of the snorkels, which were right at the bottom. Wet-weather gear, a fish smoker, smart shoes, a life jacket, bags of sawdust, more shoes, a tarpaulin, panniers, tent, crab net. How did I manage to get away with stowing such a mess? I must discover the secret of 'shipshape'. We collapsed hysterically, tight boundaries dissolving, laughing until nothing was left. Emily was fine with me then, but I can't presume today.

A cool breeze fans the morning sun across my naked belly. Mountainous coastline floats in mist, hiding the valleys. I sit in the shade of our white luminous arc. In the cool breeze, quite unexpectedly, a clear light appears inside me, growing steadily in intensity and size. It suddenly gathers me up into itself and carries me away, beyond the sea. I feel myself dissolving in the passionate embrace of the most magnificent lover ever: Life. I become the brilliant shining awareness that contains the boat, the sea, the islands. The horizon turns a misty passionate red as a fiery burning ecstasy wells up and engulfs me. Utterly surrendered, I melt into warm bubbling bliss. I become the overflowing cup. Time passes in an ordinary way, it feels like forever – maybe it is only a few minutes. Slowly I start making things more solid: the lifelines, the deck and Emily's voice calling, 'Mum, am I getting burnt?' The ecstasy of this union stays with me. I am changed. My beloved has taken me.

I stand up to break the spell and join Dad in the cockpit. *Dream-maker* is flying down the coast in the perfect breeze. Wild white breakers signal danger all along the coast.

'It's okay, Alice, I can get us in. I've been here before.'

It doesn't look okay to me. I scan the coastline for anywhere free of breaking waves. He turns *Dream-maker* towards shore.

'Dad, one of the reefing line's come loose. I can fix it.'

I jump up on deck before he can say 'no', exuberance flooding my body, and hang out over the life lines, above the swelling sea, one-footed, trusting the boom, even though it's swinging, surrendered to the moment, and throw the line out, several times, until it comes back around the end of the boom. At the navigation table with the protractor and dividers, I estimate our speed and position. I am full to the brim with the joy of sailing.

'Lunchtime,' Emily calls from the galley. The mother role always suited her best. She glows proudly, 'Here's a cup of tea for you both. I'll pass the plates up too. Here we go – fresh salad with rice and cheese.'

Dad knows the entrance through the reef into the small harbour of the Shangri-La Fijian Resort. Emily and I rush up on deck, straining to see. From a distance, the resort looks luxurious and classy. Insect-like windsurfers and little catamarans skate over the bay's surface. Green sunloafers and coconut palms line the beach. Still in our bikinis, we're ready to explore as soon as the anchor's down. Dad prises the lid off a beer. He needs to pace himself more slowly. Overarm, we slice through the warm turquoise water and introduce tanned tummies to the sunloafers and swimming pool. Emily isn't at all self conscious about our bare flesh.

'I'd love to come here for a holiday with Jack,' she dreams.

'Really! Isn't it all rather banal? There isn't an interesting-looking person in sight.'

She freezes up. She doesn't want me spoiling her world. How can she keep her own point of view when I'm like this?

I wish I could take my words back, so her face would soften again. We continue walking but I lag a little behind to stay distracted. The resort offers a kind of ordinary pleasure but I don't believe in ordinary. My heart has returned to its beloved. Our bodies are making love in every way – in the water sliding over my limbs, the tree bark poking my flesh, the wind in my face, the sand under my feet. This pleasure is extraordinary.

'Emily,' I call, to slow her down, to have us back together again, 'this holiday is so good for me. I've been given my life back. I'm in love again.'

'That's nice.' She doesn't want to know what I'm saying. She's dreaming of Jack, in a friendly, brotherly way. She doesn't want ever to fall in love after seeing what it did to me. It destroyed my life. I staggered one foot in front of the other one collapsing, all in the name love. For years I rode moments of ecstasy for months of pain. I couldn't pull out the dagger. I couldn't turn away. If she had an inkling that I've fallen in love again, what would she think then?

We continue walking, each to our own thoughts. I'm starting to understand. When I grew up, I separated out from life and from most of myself. Maybe this is what growing up means. Flying into the wind on our way here, it was like a big hand reached down to rip me open and connect us back together again. I gaze into this great wide world, my whole self – Life – bursting with love, breathing life into every moment. Whatever separates out from this breath withers and dies. Whatever separates out from this breath only pretends to be alive. I know that Emily is struggling to stay alive.

Dad welcomes us back on board *Dream-maker*. The sky fills with stars, tracing infinity. We come together for dinner under a single bulb. As I sit down, the fullness of the moment washes through me, bathing us all in a sacred, ethereal light, each moment infinitely precious. My beloved becomes the food I'm eating, the movement of my hands, the beating of my heart, full of love, bliss coursing through veins, bubbling every cell with gold. I wash dishes with the care I might wash a new born baby – each plate is only my precious beloved. We separated out so I might know him and enjoy our coming back together.

The morning is blue on blue spectacular. 'Let's check the beach out before breakfast.' I plunge into crystal clear water and bob to the surface, unable to stop the smiling, waiting for her to surface. 'Race you ashore.'

Thrashing arms torpedo us through the water, a mixture of elegance and zest, with our feet behind doing the propeller job. Our movement on shore is not so elegant, a sinking into soft sand which fortunately hardens up under the mangroves and twiggy scrub. We poke around and I take note of a small stream slipping behind the scrub. We finally splay out on the beach in bikinis, chatting with some lads.

'Time for breakfast.' I return to my normal restless and over-enthusiastic manner.

A young lad follows us into the water and starts talking to Emily, coming closer and brushing her thigh.

'No I don't want to do that,' she shouts and follows me swiftly to the boat.

A slight look of disgust stains her face. 'He must be so desperate to be touching me like this after five minutes.'

She's also excited by this other body bumping up against her.

I'm bursting with energy, but underneath … ? What am I underneath? I won't stop long enough to look. We cook up eggs and toast for a big breakfast with Dad.

'I'll stay here and sort a few things out,' he says quietly.

'Now we can explore properly. We need clothes, sandals, sunhats, water and sunscreen.'

'Okay, Mum.'

I don't give her a chance to choose something else and she doesn't mind. Doing stuff with Mum is a guaranteed adventure. What else is there to do? Dad can go ashore if he wants in the second dinghy.

I pull on the short aluminium oars and bounce us into the lagoon behind the hotel, passed a dead purple jellyfish and a couple of plastic throwaways. We manoeuvre into a narrow bayou and float through an untidy village sheltering under breadfruit and orange trees. Emily and I dispute whether a baby's cry is human or goat. We sit quietly in our own worlds, separate from each other, separate from everything outside us, just watching. A fish leaps from the water, a bird swoops in front of us, I turn us around and row back into the windy harbour.

'Where you from?' shout a group of lads at the water's edge.

'New Zealand,' Emily yells.

Their splashing turns into a Maori haka. The lads are rugby fans. Emily joins in the noise.

We row across the harbour to another shore, and beach our grey bubble boat to continue on foot, single file along the dusty track leading through scrub, past a couple of cows, to a rusting railway line and a deserted clump of buildings. There's not much to see. It's okay. We are here to see life just the way it is.

The sun is blanching everything to oblivion, including us, so we swim our boat along the shoreline to stay cool, and then set out again in search of a private sunbathing spot. Unfortunately, every clearing, small patch of sand or rocky outcrop is sprouting a lad or two with a fishing line, staring dreamily, so we head across the channel to an island.

Emily scans the shore. 'It looks deserted. We can land here.'

With our feet sucking down in the wet sand again, we lift the grey whale ashore. The sand, the beach? I'm suddenly worried about my sight because the whole beach is moving. I get it. Inside every one of the thousands of shells, is a little crab scuttling to safety. We linger over broken coral at the water's edge, then track inland looking for shelter. I lay my sarong over hard baked earth, in the shade. 'I'm going to explore.'

'I'll stay here,' Emily replies. I don't see the courage it takes for her to say so. I report back on a few roughly-weeded plots of cassava hiding inside the scrub and the occasional ant roaming the cracked ground.

'Mum, I'm tired and hungry. Let's go home.'

The wind's up and the lads across the channel watch me row against jumping waves, back out into the harbour.

'Let's sail. We can use my sarong,' I suggest. We're not making much headway against the wind.

'Okay.' Emily would put her foot down but she's too tired. I don't tend to notice when I'm tired and hungry like she is now, I'd rather have us playing my silly games. I hold one oar straight up for a mast and the other one flat for a boom. She helps tie on the sarong so the wind can blow a belly into it.

'This is great – it's working!'

'Mum. We're not moving properly. We don't have a rudder, we're sliding away from our destination.' It's so obvious.

'Oops!' I dismantle the boom and replace the oar with my arm so the oar can become a rudder for her to steer. 'We're sailing well now, sort of.'

'Mum, we're sailing in the wrong direction. We can't sail into the wind, which is the direction we want to go.' She can't help a smile now.

The lads on shore laugh. I return the oars to the water and row, momentarily chastened. The wind is still rising.

'We could row up the estuary behind the beach,' I suggest. 'It may join up with the stream we saw this morning.'

I'm happy rowing, I could row all day through the water and trees. I don't want to go home.

'Okay.' Emily's been wanting to go home for over an hour. She drifts further from a sense of who she is and what she would be doing without me. This is how we have always been.

The deep-green slow-moving estuary is beautiful with the wind gone. Large trees, arms turning down into roots, hug the water's edge. Locals crouch among the muddy roots, lines in their hands. Time passes as the oars slip us through the brackish water.

Finally Emily states the obvious: 'Mum, the estuary's taking us away from our destination. We have to turn back.'

'I know.' I turn around.

Young girls greet our return with great excitement and leap from a high tree into dark shadows of green-brown soup. I row back out into the wind and head straight for home. *Dream-maker* is empty of Dad. Emily takes off all her clothes and cruises naked into the galley to fix a cracker and cheese.

'I could be naked like you,' I laugh. 'I didn't used to be awkward about naked.'

'Course you can, Mum.'

The cool evening is delicious on our brazen flesh. Dad's buzzing outboard warns of his return. Three is one too many and I'm still restless. I hardly notice him or how he might be feeling now I have Emily. For the third time today I catch her up in my plans.

L ight from the setting sun filters through the clouds in a theatrical way. Laughing, excited and wide-eyed, we follow pathways past expensive restaurants. Apartments and shops line the exposed waterfront, dramatically accentuated against the dark night, beautiful shapes in the soft dusk. The architecture and gardens, money and aesthetics blend so well together. Why didn't I choose this kind of life?

I find Emily in a clothes store.

'Dad will be expecting dinner. We must go now.'

'The bikinis aren't that expensive,' she muses, picks out one to try on and frowns. Where's my time? Follow me for a change or at least let me do what I want?

The day comes to an end: noticing a little fish caught in the tentacles of a jelly fish and a Fijian child proud of her finely-embroidered Indian dress. I remember this day of drifting through life in a plastic dinghy. Actually I never do drift, certainly never for half an hour through racks of bikinis following my daughter.

10

I wake up, bathed in the cold sweat of a terrifying dream. It was about my son Oliver, second year studying science at University, restless and moody. In my dream he's standing all alone, clothes hanging from his thin body, feeling the burden of life, caught in the same old questions. Should I be planning for my future? Why do I always worry? Do other people like me? How can I make money? What should I be doing? Why can't I stop worrying? In that instant, without warning, an enemy sneaks up from behind and slices the top off his head. The force somersaults his body through the air, over and over as he falls slowly to the ground, totally dead, just like that – his life over.

I wake up looking death straight in the face. His death was unpredictable. Nothing in life could have saved him. Nothing in life can be depended on. I stare into infinite emptiness – the absolute finality of death, the horror, the piercing fathomless grief that must follow the death of a child. I want to shout out against the possibility, against my utter powerlessness to prevent it.

I walk outside in the morning light, into a bleached mirage. This tropical paradise, our sailing adventure, will disappear in the instant of my death, in the instant of the death of one of my children. I'm not in charge. The circumstance is uncertain, it is not worth clinging to, it is a dream and it is untrustworthy.

I don't want to build my life on sand that comes and goes with the tide. I will stay in the arms of my beloved. It doesn't matter what I do, it is all the same, it is the taste of my beloved.

I humbly follow Dad and Emily ashore, following, not leading. We cross in front of the resort stalls and their shell necklaces. Emily chats to the ladies, cross-legged on grass mats, threading beads and seeds and shells in simple patterns. Dad catches us up. I hardly see the faces or the shells. They enquire about a bus to Sigatoka.

There is nothing I want. I don't want distraction. I am nothing. As nothing I am everything. I am with my beloved. The bus rumbles away from the resort. I sit alone, gazing out the window into emerald-green countryside. Chickens scratch, leaves of sugar cane shake with the wind. I shrink from conversation that would turn me into a point of view.

At Sigatoka, Dad and Emily buy bananas and salad greens. I buy two necklaces – a string of black coral balls and a string of broken pink coral – offerings to my beloved. Around the corner, I buy two large pawpaws from a local woman who has just come from her garden. We shop and eat, kick up dust and board another bus for home.

A lemon dawn wakes up the saloon. 'Does anyone want to walk over the coral reef with me?' I have to ask. I'd rather not. 'The tide's out.'

'I'll come with you,' Dad quickly answers and puts down the coffee I just made him.

We poke around pools where teeny turquoise fish flitter, trapped until the next tide, and point to luminescent-blue starfish clinging to rocks in shapeless heaps. I find it hard to talk with Dad to bring us together. I want to slip back into the embrace of my beloved. When I was a child, he held starfish out for me to touch and helped me over slimy mudflats pocked with dangerous crab holes. I followed him into the bush and waited, gazing up buttress-rooted trees spreading splendid across the skies.

After breakfast Emily flings herself off the boat into a mayhem of water. I slip down the ladder more demurely, followed by Dad. We swim around wondering what is so great about snorkelling. I paddle over to where Dad is treading water and brush a stream of hair and water from my face.

'I'm going back to the boat. I don't want to get cold,' he says.

'Sure, we won't be long.'

He pulls down his mask and swims away, stick of snorkel zig-zagging a bee-line for *Dream-maker* and a warm beer.

I shiver from the cold in my heart and start paddling energetically around the coral gardens, following small swarms of darting fish, looking for something interesting. Emily is heading ashore. The ancient mariner is frustrated and bored, confused by his many good memories of the Shangri-La Fijian Holiday Resort. He wants a woman, a romance. I swim through swarms of poisonous sea plankton on my way to a clump of rocky coral further out. He wants to sit around talking the same old stuff I've heard a thousand times. I can't do it. I paddle faster, racing over the coral heads. I'm not going anywhere. I don't know why I'm so angry with him, but I am. I wish and wish I wasn't, but I am and I know he doesn't deserve it.

I can listen to his stories and be his human face, but not for too long. I'm trapped. My arms slap chaotically. I don't know how to stay with the discomfort of ordinary living. Swimming in the currents of my beloved, I can stay pure. I head for the beach through a shallow area buoyed off for children, safe from sharks. Another swarm of sea plankton sprays me with its poison.

Emily rolls onto her side and lifts her arm.

I have failed him. I don't want to feel guilty. My face collapses into ugly folds of guilt. I don't want this. I want to love him. What is my responsibility? I start arguing with myself and graze my knuckles on a knot of coral. I'm not responsible for his happiness. Fish and coral fade into the background. I don't know how to deal with the situation. I do have one way: I can think about it – I'm a philosopher. The water becomes shallow and my hands reach down to soft sand to pull myself to shore, paddling feet to stay afloat. I'm on familiar ground here.

Dad is responsible for his own happiness. For me to take responsibility would make less of him. My hands turn to fists in the sand. To take charge of anyone's life is an act of hatred, not love. Why am I having this conversation with myself? I stop in the water ebbing and flowing over the sand, changing light patterns. As a child I was entranced by this light. Someone took me away from it, again and again. Someone told me who I was, how I should be, what I should do. No one cared about me. This was my life growing up. I plead some more with my hard heart. I know there isn't any other way. Belly down on wet sand, belly covered in white glitter standing up.

Emily rolls onto her back and covers her face with a sarong. 'Mum, am I getting burned anywhere? Can you rub some sunscreen on my moles?'

Children snorkel in the cordoned-off area while their mothers watch from sun-loafers and the coconut palms whisper encouragement to their green nuts. I lie on my stomach, head in my hands, and stare into the grains of sand – hard rock weathered into soft powder. Dad is lonely, the cussed adventurer is old, life tricked him. He walks into each day with his shoulders stooped, looking down. He has lost the power of a new dream.

Night arrives early. We sit all shrunken up in the cockpit, distracted by fruit bats flying to the mainland. Unsettled birdsong tinkles over the mirrored surface of the sea. A fog of gloomy resentment fills the air. I ask about the bats. The night is warm, but I start to shiver. I don't know what's going on between us. We never talk about how we feel, so how could I? I stare blankly at my feet and Dad takes out a cigarette and gazes blankly into space.

Resentment was the poison in our family. I don't know who the whiff I'm getting now belongs to. Mum and Dad expected to be happy in their marriage. Their unspoken disappointment steamed and composted into a chilly resentment. The sixties arrived just in time to save them. They slid down the rabbit hole of encounter groups and learned that it was okay to smile and scream and be happy. Dad gave up the misery of trying to be good. He grabbed hold of his life and went sailing. I left home as soon as I could. Pockets of resentment still flare up. One day I will be free of them – then I can stay in the ordinary world.

Emily climbs up into the cockpit and snuggles next to me. 'Mum, let's go back ashore and dance. There's a disco tonight.'

Music wafts enticingly across the water from the hotel.

'What!' I start. 'I can't remember the last time I went dancing.'

'Come on, I don't want to go on my own.'

She pulls at my arm like an impatient child.

"Well, I have to admit you do what I want most of the time. I can pretend to be young and silly.'

She leads me downstairs to dress up. Our hair is stiff with salt.

'It's funny, Mum. I feel pretty until I try to make myself look pretty – then I feel plain.'

'You look lovely.'

We follow the music upstairs into a large bar and start shaking around on the dance floor.

An Australian golfer comes across to our table. 'Would you like to dance?'

'Sure.' I squirm with the pleasure of being noticed.

He's slightly bald on top, grey around the edges, hair probably dyed, not much of a gut, quite presentable in a very ordinary way, here for a week at a golfing tournament.

After a couple of dances he leans forward, 'Would you like to get laid?'

I laugh. 'Why, thank you, but no, that's not quite my style.'

Relaxing in the shadows, Emily asks, 'Do you think Jack and I will be together?'

I have a split second to make a choice. 'Well, to be perfectly honest, I don't think you are similar enough, so probably not.'

The pink in Emily's cheeks turns grey. She never should have asked and I realise in that moment that I shouldn't have answered.

'You wanted me to marry Paul, didn't you?' She persists, angry with herself for continuing. It doesn't matter what Mum thinks, she can make her own choices. She waits for the answer, already crying inside.

'I liked Paul,' I tentatively reply.

'But he was so controlling, he kept telling me what to think.' He face becomes contorted, almost ruined. 'I tried to be like him and I was so miserable. When we broke up I had no idea who I was any more. Jack lets me be myself.'

'You seemed pretty miserable in Fiji with him.'

'I know. I don't know what's wrong with me.'

Dad wants to leave for Musket Cove, a yachtie haven on Malolo Lailai Island, a little further up the coast.

'Dad, I don't want to leave yet.' He doesn't look up. 'We're starting to make friends. I like getting to know a new place.'

I turn to Emily for support. She doesn't care.

'We can't be too long away from Lautoka,' he replies coldly. 'We need to check in with customs there because we're in a different part of Fiji now.'

We motor into a head wind without putting up the sails. They'd flap uselessly. The engine grumbles below, a noisy smelly thrust pushing us through the choppy sea. After several hours of bumping and thrashing, we turn into a narrow channel between the main island and its reef and finally win our destination, Musket Cove. Dick Smith, the local developer, has crowded the bay with large mooring buoys for rent. We anchor further out. Dad bundles us all into the dinghy and putters ashore, fingers crossed that our spirits will revive in the convivial atmosphere of the 'three dollar bar'. A bulldozed breakwater provides marina-type facilities for those willing to pay. Dad leads the way across a small bridge, with side rails to stop the drunkards falling in, and along a spit of reclaimed land to the crowning glory, 'the two dollar bar', recently renamed 'the three dollar bar.' The good anchorage, the bar, the modern shower block and a store selling chicken and sausages for the barbecue bring in boaties from all over the world.

Barbecues, roaring with wood supplied by management, fill the environs with the rich smell of burning fat. Emily and I hover on the sandy floor under brightly-coloured light bulbs while Dad orders rum. Casually-dressed rough-whiskered single-handers drink at the bar. The women, sparsely spread, tend the food. I follow Emily as she throws herself cheerfully into conversation. Dad hands drinks around. I rattle my glass mindlessly. I don't want to be here. I open a seedling coconut with a single-hander looking for company. His much younger girlfriend left years ago to return to college. We taste the cheesy 'bread' and share it round. Dad throws back rums at the bar with a seventy-one-year-old Irishman, who took up sailing when he was sixty-five and boasts a single-handed run from England to New Zealand in a small Warrum catamaran.

I was bitten by thousands of poisonous plankton at Shangri-La. Blood, pus, salt and sweat crust over the angry wounds. Next morning Emily and I row ashore and head for the large bathroom: white-tiled floor, smooth tiled walls, large polished mirrors. We stand forever under large stainless shower heads, shampooing and soaping and shaving and, for me, cleaning off my grubby sores.

'I'll find my own way back to the boat,' Emily says gaily when we dump our towels and shampoo in the dinghy. She's meeting a couple of young backpackers on the beach. I set out along the main path – grey cloud rolling overhead, grey cloud rumbling inside – past clusters of resorts, around a golf course, through a private airstrip, onto a peninsular of mown coconut plantations. This whole island has been made over for middle-class pleasure. I stomp into the hard dust. Where are the grass houses and simple fishermen and colourful strings of washing and dark-skinned youths splashing in the water?

I sit on the hillside above Musket Cove, following the turquoise-green necklace around the island. Coral lies just under the surface of the water – treacherous if you're trying to sail over it, beautiful if you're swimming through it. Dark choppy ocean stretches to the horizon. I've reefed all my sails and locked myself up. Dad wants to keep moving. I'm resisting. I'm not being contrary – I don't like it here, but I need to be in one place for more than a night or two, even this ghastly place.

When I encountered my beloved, sailing up the coast, he propelled me into a new body. His fiery embrace opened me up to a different kind of sensing. I'm losing this sensing. I discovered the same kind of sensing when I was cycling around East Cape. I was neither separate from nor the same as fragile butterflies and fragrant spring blossom. Then I came to realise how fundamentally I depend on sensing – the finer the sensing, the richer the world. 'Sensing' was one of those words like 'memory' and 'time' that I had always taken for granted. Maybe it's the most important word of all. Without it, 'world' and 'me' are impossible. Maybe there's nothing but sensing. I sense objects, thoughts, mental images, feelings, movement, the development of thought. Take away sensing and you take away me and every possible world I could live in.

I imagine building myself out of Lego, different coloured blocks representing information from different senses. Yellow builds me and my world up from the sounds of my voice, the sound of the sea; white from the smells of seaweed, the smell of my sweat; blue from the colour of my hair, the sight of the morning sun; red from all the feeling qualities – solid, heavy, soft – inside and on my skin.

I imagine taking my senses away. All the white pieces of smelling go, then the yellow pieces of hearing, the blue pieces of seeing and the yellow ones of sound. I can hold on for a while to the thinning skeleton, filling in the gaps mentally. Then it's all gone, I only have memory. Memory is a kind of sensing, a mental sensing. That goes as well – no mental images. Then I start hallucinating myself and other people into reality. Then I go mad. It was a gobsmacking discovery for me as an adult to realise just how important sensing is. We sense ourselves and our worlds into existence. The finer the sensing, the richer the world.

My new way of sensing builds a finer world as a layer behind the ordinary one. In this world I'm like a child – I haven't separated out: I'm embodied in my experience. I want this world back. I'm angry that the grown-ups should have taken me away from it. The finer the sensing, the more slowly I need to move. I can't skate over the surface of life in a windsurfer while I swim deep ocean currents of bliss. I need to move slowly if I want to ride the wind, not as it rushes past my face but as it stirs me gently inside, if I want to notice a different light in every bay, if I want to become as fine as a grain of pollen on the wind. I want this.

That's it. I stand up indignantly and glare at the threatening clouds. This is my fight. This is what I could never accept about ordinary living. It's a conspiracy that keeps us distracted from ourselves, from life. I wonder if the yachties at the three dollar bar ever let go the already known. Do they ever get naked enough to be impressed by anything new? Their lives have been forfeited. Doesn't anyone know what's happening? I want to scream. The clouds roll and crackle above me. We trade in our courage for someone else's hand-me-downs. I want to tell my father that life only breathes in the present moment; he won't find it in his mansion of memories.

I walk slowly down from the summit, back through the resorts and along the breakwater. Sometimes I wonder if it's me that got life wrong. Trouble is I don't know what to do with this kind of wondering. It's too late to change my course. I can fine-tune my sail but I can't change my course. I can't return to a conventional life.

A morning swim clears my head. Cigarette smoke pours out the companionway and I dress in the cockpit, watching boats, planes and helicopters carrying tourists back and forth from the mainland.

Dad comes out. 'Alice, I've been thinking. I want to stay in Fiji until the end of September. The family can come over and visit us here.' He looks angry – he knows I'm going to fight him.

I whip around. 'Dad, that's four months from now. This wasn't our plan. I thought you'd given it up.'

'Well, I've changed my mind. It makes sense to stay.'

'What sense? We won't have any time to visit anywhere else. That's not fair. It's not what we agreed to. I don't want to spend my whole six months in Fiji sitting in harbours. I want an adventure. I need to move slowly, that's all.'

I can't see that Dad is lonely. My fine mystical realm doesn't include him – it protects me from him.

Dream-maker isn't my favourite place this morning. Last night we went ashore again to eat. I can't stand it when my mind crashes into the conventional and tosses around in gravel kicked up by passing cars. My beloved has gone. I'm not happy in this shrunken pretence. A hundred boats huddle together in the harbour, weighed down by vanity and money, stealing the space, shutting out the light. I'm cynical. Boats are meant to be the wings of freedom and adventure. Here, smooth-running engines carry well-heeled passengers from one harbour to the next. This was the lie that killed me when I was young. These boats are comfortable statements of ordinary mind, safely tethered. Their well-stayed masts assert an unassailable self-importance.

There's nothing wrong with boats in a harbour. The day is grey and windy. Alone on the boat, I stop my writing and make a hot drink. Dad returns with his washing and Emily's on shore with her new friends. I go ashore to walk, eyes bleary and strained. I need a

lonely place to meditate and open myself up again. I walk and walk;
I sit up, lie down, but still my mind stays tight. I walk again. What's
to be done? I can't do anything. Suddenly, in the gap between lifting
one foot and putting it down, the dream of Oliver's death flashes
before me; the certainty of death lands on my shoulder and wakes
me up into the present moment. Through the eyes of death I see the
fleeting irretrievable nature of every moment.

My eyes soften in the return of my beloved. The ordinary becomes
radiant and beautiful. I walk down to the beach on the other
side of the island. Here the washed up plastic bottles and bags are
placed to perfection. The strong winds roaring on the side I came
from are gone. Here the sea is clear and still. Under young wattle and
small red-leafed shrubs, on the soft damp ground, I shape a matted
cushion of twigs and leaves with my sarong neatly on top. Prickly-
seeded plants and arching, flowering grasses shape the melting air.
I fill with the finest pleasure, my heart melts into the perfection of
everything. If the yachties knew how overwhelmingly fine it is to be
like this, wouldn't they want to find a way? Maybe they would be
scared of such orgasmic pleasure, scared of giving themselves up,
scared of losing themselves utterly. They would rather pretend to be
happy with a beer and roasted pig.

I wake early from the arms of my love, hostility pounding in my
ears. I want to strangle Dad. He picks and needles. He puts me into
a box he won't let me out of. He won't live his own life. He latches
onto me, concerned, resentful, interested, judging. He comments on
everything I do. When I talk with him, I become nothing – an unreal
projection of his – so I don't. I become sullen, introverted, despondent
and unconfident, the way I was as a child. We set sail for Lautoka
after another ridiculous exchange about plans. He won't be straight
about what he wants and just grumbles about what he thinks I want.

11

The mainland arrives as a rugged sleepy animal, too big for empire builders to obliterate. People crawl over her back, shelter in her valleys and plant grain on the plains. She's bigger than all of them.

I sit outside with my morning coffee to gaze upon our new watery Lautoka home – an expansive glassy harbour with only three other yachts, softly faded in the distance. Protective arms of scrubby land shelter us from the unpredictable sea. Nearby, a rusty watchtower shell leans precariously over the water, its pokey windows glance anxiously to the jetty on shore, also slip-sliding, rotting, collapsing into the sea. Voices from shore fade behind broken birdsong and the noise of our sail sliding across itself on the rocking boom. In the shivering water, the rising sun turns small dwellings at the water's edge into tall multi-levelled skyscrapers. The top layers break the laws of gravity and tumble into the sky like giant seabirds. A purple jellyfish pulses through the water in frilly pink bellbottoms.

Emily and I walk the back streets into Lautoka, which is as Indian as Suva is Fijian. We trudge up one main street and down the other, remarking on the tidy row of colonial palms and the railway line, abstracting a mind map so we don't get lost. We joke about how the clothes shops sell pots and pans and hardware stores sell food. The food looks terrible and tastes terrible. In a Chinese restaurant selling boiled taro and cassava, I pick at oily over-cooked chicken and unburden myself.

'I need to talk about Dad. I don't want to, but I'm desperate.'

'Sure, I'll listen. I know you don't want me to take sides.'

'Dad's seventy-seven. He's old. He doesn't have the energy for new adventures. For him, this trip is a mistake.' I pause to disentangle myself from my emotions. 'I'm going crazy,' I confess. 'I can't stand being around him. I'm being strangled.' I fall into desperation. 'I want to scream all the time. It's not his fault.' I say this but I don't believe it. I'm trying to be fair. 'Something has to change.'

I've carried time bombs of 'wanting to scream all the time' and 'feeling strangled' into all my relationships with men.

'Well, Mum, what do you suggest?' She understands exactly what I'm saying. She could be having this conversation about me and I know it.

'I need to get away. That's all I can do. Let's go away for a couple of weeks?'

'Sure, Jack and I didn't see much. It would be fun.' Mum is fun most of the time.

'I hate being like this. Forget about it all now. It's nothing to do with you, okay?' I try another forkful of limp noodles. 'There's nothing wrong with Dad. I know that. It's about me.'

'Don't worry, I'm enjoying the holiday.' Grandad seems perfectly normal to her.

We leave our half-eaten meals and difficult conversation and head for the market, stopping at some clothes shops on the way.

'Look, Mum, a bag of Australian clothes for $1. Let's go inside.'

'Long-sleeved silk shirts for sailing,' I call after her. We flick through racks of too many shorts, tops and shirts. Emily strips down to knickers and bra, behind a rack, while I keep watch and pass the garments one by one. Modest young shop assistants smile indulgently.

We're back in our old happy roles. At another shop, we ask about prickly fruit and Indian gods sitting by the pots and pans.

'Ganesh the elephant removes obstacles,' a serious young lad informs us. 'You find him outside all the temples.'

We continue on, checking the different shops, up and down the two main streets. Our dinghy is parked near the derelict remainder of a marina, destroyed in a cyclone before it was finished, now waiting for a new idea. The night watchman points to a muddy, grimy tiled box. Cold water pours straight from a pipe. Fijian workers shower here. I tingle with excitement. Life is only just holding on. This is real, how life actually is. A corroded pipe, tied up with wire is honest, no deception, teetering on dissolution, no illusion of permanence, purely functional. Life is always teetering on dissolution. My mother was like this, always teetering on disillusion and dissolution.

'Mum, you'll have to stand guard. There's no door. Hold my clothes. I'll go first.'

'Don't you love doing this kind of thing?'

'I do. I know what you mean.' She hangs out with her mum to feel alive.

I'm needing to get back to the bare basics, to start again so I can grow strong and true. 'Emily, which do you prefer, this shower or the ones at Musket Cove?'

'Mmm ... I like both of them. I didn't mind Musket Cove.' She falters under the falling water. Why does Mum have to compare them? Why does she hate luxury so much?

My turn with cold water pouring down through my hair and I decide to hate the showers at Musket Cove. Too middle-class, a symbol of money, easy comfort and consumer values. Who's angry – the waif who couldn't find a home there or the insightful spiritual renegade?

'We have to pick up our emails. There may be one from Jack.'

She hurries me along as I linger to look around. Next to each other in front of our computer screens, we wait forever for each page to download.

'A letter from Jack! He's fine and he's missing me.' She has her own life again, her dream of a man.

'That's nice. I'm still waiting on my computer.' My anxiety rises. I feel trapped, tied to the chair. I can't escape my fate. Finally the letters download.

James wants to come over for a holiday, but I doubt he will. The roof at Orere is leaking in five places while Trish, my friend and tenant, patiently moves buckets and furniture until I sort it.

Girlfriends and sisters are warm and chatty. My other children, Charlotte and Oliver, are studying and sound happy and keen to come sailing if Dad and I roam further afield than the Pacific, which I doubt we will. I forget I have friends and family. I can't hold onto them because I'm too panicky inside. I close down the computer. It's over, I survived. I glow, remembering my life back home.

In the night, I dream of building a little thatch hut for myself in the bush, far away from the city. I paint the window frames bright fresh colours with the help of three nieces and my three children. My three hens lay ten eggs on their first morning. I need this simple dream, my mind is so tied up in knots at the moment.

A big tidy up of the boat would help. I retrieve clothes, oils, bags and shoes dropped all over the place. The jumble of clothes in my locker and bunk resembles my son's bedroom at its worst. Dad's up on deck fixing something. When he comes downstairs for tools I can tell he's happy, because he has a problem he can solve. Emily stretches out on her bunk, rocked gently by the ocean swell, lost in her book. I wipe over the galley and then sit down in the cockpit to drift away into memories.

Memories of the relationship I left behind. We're all dreaming of romance on this boat. He's never far away, this man of flesh and blood, the man I took into my heart for ten tumultuous years, the man I could neither live with nor live without. He's a huge unsorted mess inside me. I didn't know how to start on the mess, so I sailed away from him. In my memory we stand on opposite sides of an abyss, into which a light never shined, into which we fell, over and over.

I prefer the good memories today, the ones that make my heart sing. We'd fly by helicopter into the Kawekas, raw and wild, mist covered mountains. We dragged deer carcasses up the scrubby faces with the night rolling in, and wrapped up together in a small tent, alone in the great wilderness. I fell in love with the mountains, the wild weather and with him. I never separated them out. I never understood why our tender life-affirming embraces turned into angry destructive rages. He's a long way away now, but I keep him in my heart, to have someone there.

My head starts throbbing inside an iron cage that's crushing me. I stagger down to my bunk. I am not used to these headaches. They were a constant part of my childhood, but they stopped in my thirties when I became a meditating yogi. They have returned. I stop thinking, swallow some Paracetamol and rest, eyes tight shut. By afternoon it's over and a brand new mind emerges, a soft open mind.

'Emily, shall we go ashore for a bit and walk?'

She glances up, all mellowed out by her romance, legs restless in the heat.

'Sure. I'll finish my chapter – give me ten minutes.'

The tide is out, exposing a rugby field of mud between us and shore. I know the impossibility of plodding through soft squelchy mud dragging a dinghy. It's not an option. Emily would turn back.

'We'll use the jetty.'

'The ladder's five feet out of the water.' She remembers the sarong sailing fiasco. Here we go again!

I motor the laden dinghy alongside, bumping against the soft slimy poles.

'Okay, you go first.'

Emily hauls herself up the slimy and then dry rungs, surprising herself with the fun of it. The mud on her clothes will brush off when it dries.

I pass up the packs and empty jerry cans one by one, then loop my arm through the side arm of the ladder and swing up quite elegantly, holding onto the painter.

'Now we have to haul the dinghy up.' It looks impossible to Emily. The outboard motor is heavy. We pull together, inch by inch – small progress is all we need. Together we can do it, ten feet all the way up. It's good when there's no other option but to keep going. At last the grey belly flops over onto the jetty like a beached seal.

'That's it. See, it was easy,' I beam with exaggerated delight.

Emily smiles back, slightly irritated with the game.

We stroll past fibrolite homes tucked under breadfruit trees. Leaves decorate the raked earth. In the cool afternoon I take her arm like a child and follow, enjoying how blissful and simple my mind is now. Sailing into Lautoka the other day, Emily had remarked that she was in an utterly blissful place – everything seemed perfect. I'm in that place now, quiet and open, nothing required. Young people gather for the evening. We linger outside a mosque at the back of town, the streets fill with families on their way to church. Hymns pour from open doors on every corner, enticing the stragglers.

I return to our dinghy ahead of Emily, to walk alone in this soft mind. Black smoke from a Pacific liner hangs motionless in the blue-on-blue stillness of sky. Couples stroll the jetty and brightly-painted fishing boats hang at anchor. Everything is vivid in the cool dusk light. A young Indian woman approaches, followed by her boyfriend, and then a Fijian couple with their two children. Emily arrives. I excuse myself from their inquisitive conversation to lug our heavy cans of water along the jetty, steady as it lurches from side to side because some of the poles have rotted away.

Our dinghy flops easily into a full tide. I start the motor once we're away from the rotting poles. The sea is glassy. The full moon begins its rise over the horizon. Guitar melodies arouse singing, stomping and clapping all around town.

'Mum, I'm thinking I might only stay another couple of weeks.'

Perfect eternity disappears instantly. I turn both hot and cold, in quick succession. The outboard motor suddenly stops.

'Really, that's not very long.' I try to sound casual but my voice is thin and high- pitched .

'No, but I'm missing Jack.'

I pull the starting cord. The motor starts briefly, then it stops.

'Well, we'll have time to go away, at least,' I squeak.

I pull again, with a little more tension. The engine starts and we continue on course. Of course my life will continue after she's gone. I can leap the swamp of loss when she leaves. Maybe I've been rushing her around too much, catching her up in my plans. I don't know how to do it differently.

'Hi, Dad. We're back. I'll cook dinner now. Sorry we're a bit late.'

He looks up from his whiskey and turns down the radio. His whiskers bristle. 'I wanted to go in and watch the rugby up at the Northerner. Now it's too late.' He shuffles off, looking for his cigarettes. He's been on his own all afternoon while we've been in town. He didn't say anything about rugby to me. I dismiss his grizzling. The weight of responsibility in my headache is gone. Grumpy, happy or otherwise, he can deal with it. I fall asleep to melodic, soulful hymns soaring low across the water.

12

I need to calm down, reef my sail, meditate. Cross-legged in the saloon with a cushion in the small of my back, I sink under my tumbling thoughts, through my compulsive activity, behind the entrancing glamour of living. I follow my breath slowly down into a still clear well of just knowing, deep within. I bare myself to a love that is waiting, a full embrace. I embody a quality of intelligence I can barely withstand. I know that all things are as they should be in this most perfect of worlds. The whole of life is living me. I don't need to hold on. What I have is worth much more. When I resurface, I'm clear and calm again.

As we do every day, Emily and I set off for town to walk the streets, up and down and up and down, filling in time before a movie. Somewhere I'm scared that, if I stop, I will fall into a hollow dreadful emptiness that isn't the waiting room of love. I will fall into a lonely, cold hole of nothing. Lugging bags of shopping, legs tired, back aching, I drop into a comfy seat next to Emily in the picture theatre. The bright Technicolor screen takes over our minds and we disappear into another world. What a relief! Emily passes the popcorn and folds her legs up on the seat.

'What did you think of David Gray's definition of fantasy in the movie?' I ask afterwards, as we start heading back to the boat.

'I don't remember. What did he say?'

'He said it right at the beginning, when he was teaching philosophy to the kids at college.' Emily shrugs and turns back to a shop window, fixing on the gold-threaded pattern in a sari. 'Our fantasies are dreams we don't want to come true. We hold onto them to escape our lives. One minute we're in our lives, the next we're lost in fantasy.'

Pretty blouses and skirts hang from plastic dummies. 'We want real dreams to come true, we work at them, they happen slowly,' I add, trying to get clear for myself what the difference is.

Emily replies, 'I don't know what my dreams are. My only real dream is to have a family. It's not enough.' She pauses. 'What's important is how I live each day. That's all I've really got.'

What! Did she discover this for herself or hear it from me?

'I agree.' We walk on quietly for a bit. 'You and I are so different. I keep drowning in life, hurling myself at everything, finding it all so interesting. You're always uncertain what to do. You resist, you often won't even try.'

'It doesn't seem worth it. I can't watch life if I'm caught up in it? How will I know if I'm doing okay?' She hesitates. 'I'm scared to let go. I need to check on what I'm doing. Maybe I'll get it wrong. It's true. I'm scared of losing control.'

We walk without talking for a couple of minutes. My steps are quick, Emily's are slow and long.

She continues, 'There's something else. I don't want to be the person who's a teacher or anything else, because that person isn't all the other things I want to be. I can't be them all. I don't know how to choose.'

I turn to face her. ' And once we've chosen a role, society takes us over.'

'I have these voices inside my head, judging me. I'm so scared of getting it wrong. Where do they come from?'

'I have them too. I don't know. I don't know how people live. Ordinary life doesn't make sense to me.' I rush off at a tangent. 'Surely we are here to experience life? Desire drives living. It threw you into Jack's arms. It brought us to Fiji. Our desire for happiness is driving this conversation.'

'You're not making sense.'

My thoughts race ahead. I don't stop to explain myself. We're still walking vaguely in the direction of the boat.

'Desire reduces awareness. You want to know and I want to experience. I want both. They're enemies. I threw my spiritual books down on the horns of this dilemma. How can we live an uncommitted, aware life? You are trying and it doesn't work, does it? Why would we want to?' I pause, only for breath. 'The Buddha talked about giving up attachment, giving up desire.'

I spin around, frustrated and freed at how clearly this doesn't make sense. 'Without attachment, which is the nature of every relationship we have, we wouldn't exist. Don't you see?'

I glare at Emily as if she were responsible for the problem.

'Without attachment and desire I have no way of living my life, of belonging. What could the Buddha have possibly meant? His freedom seems like a freedom from existing, from every possibility of happiness. Life's incredible. It's for living, not rejecting. Jesus talked about fulfilling life. There must be another way. Stop, let me think about this.'

We stand under a street light, in the dark. Emily breathes in the sultry air, eyes following the few passersby, and waits. My face lights up again.

'Somehow we aren't fully present in our lives, we have never totally accepted our human birth and the world it made for us. That's what I think.'

'Accepted our human birth?' Her eyes go dull as she turns away. 'Wait ... ' She turns back. 'I do see what you mean. I'm always resisting. I resist getting involved and I dream of Jack to escape. It's not like we have a good time together. That's amazing. I don't accept my life. I'm scared.' She bubbles at this possible solution to her dilemma.

I continue: 'I throw myself into activity. I'm unstoppably busy. You resist. You stay on shore and watch. Neither of us has an answer. We're both escaping life.'

'I don't understand how you can be so into the spiritual life and then do stupid things like fall in love with Max.' She withdraws into herself. 'I don't live easily, I wish I knew what I was meant to be doing. I know I feel tired all the time because I don't know what to do.'

Next day we bus to a concrete bus stop in the interior highlands of Fiji to sit in its concrete shade, out of the dusty heat, sharing a bottle of water. Wild seedlings of eggplant, pawpaw and guava grow through the long grass. We move with the sun, closer to the shady end and away from the ants. We don't talk much. Homes shelter under rocky bluffs, surrounded by modest vegetable gardens, sugar cane plantations, fruit trees and a few animals. Emily and I dream of this way of life. When it gets cooler, we walk along the road to its end. A young lad in a freshly-pressed white shirt and oiled hair is waiting for the bus. A group of scruffy young children head towards us carrying small fishing rods. The late bus drops us back in Lautoka.

Between mouthfuls of lukewarm chow mein, I start another conversation. 'I've been thinking about habits, how they take over our lives.' I stuff another forkful of noodles into my mouth. 'We should be worried about how what we know controls us, rather than worrying about what we don't know. We think we live in fear of what we don't know, when it isn't the real problem.' I speak slowly and clearly. 'It's what we know that kills us, not what we don't know.'

Emily is bored enough to have a go at following my new idea. 'That's such a complicated way of saying it. You mean that we have to break through what we know, to keep growing, to stay alive.'

'Wow, you've got it! We regurgitate the known over and over. Like the tree, most of us is dead wood.'

'Mum, you can't be that judgemental. How do you know?'

We head for a café that sells chocolate cake and coffee. 'That's why Dad is so difficult. He's lost in his habits. Everything he does or says is predictable. The boat is claustrophobic.'

'I haven't noticed. I don't have much to do with him.'

Under the chocolate icing on my face, my thoughts race on.

'Our willingness to stand in the unknown, in the unpredictable flow of life, returns us to ourselves. The present is unknown, it's a place of great power, beyond control and judgement and way beyond voices in our head telling us how to behave.'

Emily leaps with me to get a glimpse, a magnificent taste of freedom.

'I just understand. That's so cool.'

We start back to the boat, spilling with ideas. The night is bursting with electricity, alive with power, full of a thousand possibilities. What we've discovered is so contrary to normal thinking, it's so clever. The logic is clear, Emily thinks, so maybe it's true.

'Let's write it down so we don't forget.' She hunts for pen and paper. Under the neon light of a gas station she scribbles down our statement of our freedom:

We've discovered that the known is the enemy. That's what's scary. We need courage to return to the boat and succumb to its life-threatening habits and all-consuming routines. To the known we must return.

We burst into laughter at the turnaround. As children, the known was a source of comfort. We were scared of the unknown, weren't we? What changed? Emily continues to write as I expound:

What is all this bullshit about fear of the unknown? It's the known that does you in. Go live your dreams before your habits outlive you.

We keep producing grand statements.

Life is unknown, the cutting edge of the known penetrating the unknown. We agree with Marx – we have nothing to lose but our chains.

We start giggling as the import of our insight penetrates. We can't stop breaking into laughter as we surrender to the power, the rushing stream of endless possibility. We can't hold onto any of it, and keep collapsing into deepening whirlpools of fun, spinning us together. We're more than our habits, we can see freedom, we can win now we know the enemy.

Maybe we were just totally worn out from walking the main street seven times after spending most of the day in the hills? We keep spilling all the way to the wharf and into the dinghy, through the waves, softening and exposing ourselves. Every idea that comes up, we unmask with lighthearted ridicule. We unearth the rabbit-hole hiding places of everyone we know, exposing their strategies for keeping safe in the known, laughing uproariously at our cleverness. How we hide behind the known! Poor Dad, he doesn't stand a chance. It doesn't stop when we climb onboard. We are only momentarily chastened by his helpless seriousness.

Tomorrow we leave to backpack around the island. Packs, tent, cooker and bed mats tumble out into the saloon. The boat bubbles with our brightly-coloured plans. Still caught in the swirling dance of hysteria, we are like warm bottles of coke accidentally opened and there's no way to put the fizz back inside. When our packs are full and strapped tightly down, we go to bed. Sleepless, too emptied-out to need sleep, I wake early, clear and buoyant. Dad is understandably perfunctory and annoyed, he's become an outsider on his own boat.

He motors us, finally subdued, to the marina at Vuda Point, where he'll stay while we're away.

'Bye, Dad. Have a good rest while we're away. Hope you meet some nice people.' I give him a short hug.

'I'll be fine,' he grunts.

An American sailor on the boat next door watches us leave. He decides to stay there until we return.

PART THREE

13

Our packs bulge with everything we might need, even though we don't know where we're headed or what we're going to do.

I hoist the rugged carcass up on my back, and settle into the weight, memories, sense of freedom. We belong together. 'I love this.'

'I'm the same.' Emily smiles at me.

We board a bus heading north and settle comfortably into our own worlds, quiet as can be. The bus rattles through the countryside, through small villages, along the broken coastline. Emily leans into the window frame, floating away in dreams of Jack, remembering her friends in Golden Bay.

The Indian bus driver and ticket collector chat, gesticulating back and forth, in stops and starts, with the bus. Their bright, animated faces look forward into bright futures. Pop music blasts above the engine roar as an incoherent, noisy mush.

'Mum, I recognise the music. It's Eminem and J-Lo.' She follows the melody for a few lines then drifts away.

Well-dressed Indians with thickly-oiled hair climb aboard at every stop. Today the sugar-cane harvest began. Although most of the plantations belong to the Indians, rough-shirted Fijians machete the vast plantations, one cane at a time. Heavily-laden carts creep along the road.

'The countryside is so beautiful.' We both stare out the window, caught by the golden rolling hills.

'I can imagine living here,' Emily replies dreamily. Golden-brown grass catches afternoon light. 'Look at that little house over there, under the hill, with its garden. I could bring my children up there. It's like Orere.'

The sea re-appears, feeding mangroves, inlets and sandy beaches. A solitary person here, a small family group there, stand by the roadside as we pass.

I settle back into myself, to meditate – opening out my mind to look directly at the thoughts and images making me up. I don't become absorbed in my thoughts in an ordinary way, like Emily is now. Instead, I study them like one might study different coloured threads in a patterned mat. I like to see what they are – flickering images of consciousness – where they have come from, and how they got woven into my mat. I like doing this, to be become free of myself and feel spacious, without boundaries, without definition.

It suddenly dawns on me that I am a person, only because others know me and tell me to be myself. This clarity feels like an original discovery. Don't I already know this? I sit up straight, to see more clearly into the matter. There is no independent, autonomous Alice sitting on this bus seat. I am a story that has been shaped by others and by my genes. I'm a social and biological phenomenon. There is nothing I can find in all my thinking and memories that is original. Not only that, all my thoughts are just thoughts. They don't exist in the world. Who I think myself to be doesn't exist outside my mind. That's a sobering realisation that doesn't seem to relate to my ordinary life.

Our bus approaches Rakiraki, the northernmost town of Viti Levu. I stand up and wriggle about, to recreate my solid body, and walk up the aisle, noisily, so the driver will notice me.

'Excuse me. Is there a place we can camp for the night or is there a backpackers?'

His white teeth smile as his forehead bumps up in thought: 'Nooo.' He thinks some more and then smiles all over again. 'You can camp in the police compound. You'll be safe there. There's nowhere else.'

He turns away and then back when I ask for directions. 'Wait till we get there. I'll take you.'

At the police station, we grab our packs and follow him in. The officer in charge keeps shaking his head without looking at us. 'It will be noisy. It would be most unusual.' The Indian bus driver talks heatedly in Fijian until the officer nods. 'That's fine. Come, I'll show you around.' He smiles and points to the front lawn on the noisy main road. 'Sometimes the night watchmen get drunk. It can get pretty noisy.'

'Thank you so much. We won't be any trouble. We're happy to use the toilets at the market and to get water from there.' I haven't seen the market toilets.

A small group of police officers gather to laugh and joke, watching us put up the tent.

After a few minutes huddled inside, hot and sticky, Emily grabs the daypack. Closing the gate behind, we wave goodbye to the officers. Down the road music pours from the local church. We keep walking. Islamic declarations to God arrive with dusk. We walk to the outside of town and back. Now in the twilight, soulful Fijian love songs float from shadowy alcoves and pour into the night. We keep walking – there's nothing else to do.

In the dark, zippered safely from inquisitive mosquitoes, we sprawl out in our tent – naked, limbs helplessly overheating, the single flame of a candle lantern flickering. Cars, utes and trucks grumble noisily down the main street. Excited, volatile conversation fills the air. Deep voices angrily cut through a softer, placating female chatter. The violent volcanic energy that gave birth to these islands lies just beneath the surface.

Morning light filters through the emerald tent fly as I wrestle free of a twisted sheet.

'Emily, are you awake?' She doesn't move. 'What a night!' I sit up and grab the water bottle. 'The officer in charge warned us: "The night watchmen drink a lot of kava. They can party all night." He was right. What about the trucks!'

Emily rolls over sleepily. 'I think I slept through most of it.'

I groan, hanging from my shoulders. 'I don't know if I can face another day in a bus. I'm totally shattered.'

I open the tent fly and peek out into a town waking up with us. Like a child, sleep still in my eyes, I start down to the market toilets, not smelling or looking around. Broadcasted Islamic chanting blasts me totally awake.

We dismantle the tent and head to the river for breakfast.

'Here, Mum.' She hands me a bowl of oats soaked in fresh milk, sliced banana on top. On the grassy river bank I mix yeast, spirulina and kelp into two glasses of water. The river is a cloudy, stationary ooze. Rubbish and tree debris pile up on its banks, waiting for a good rain. Sun sparkles the muddy surface. A fella picks at rubbish with a rake and shovel. The seats are broken and someone's hosing the toilets. A pretty pathetic adventure. Already I'm barely surviving. Emily walks away down to the river to eat alone.

I meditate to sweep my mind clean and arrive back in the present moment. Meditation is always a good solution to unacceptable situations. Now, through new eyes the day swells full through the soaring chants, exclaiming the vans, the ambulance on the bridge, pigeons wheeling and cooing, townsfolk busy with another day. A thin blade of grass uncurls and a small flower turns to the sun. I feel the exhaustion of being forever trapped in this churning and stirring, ravelling and unravelling, utterly empty activity.

A dewdrop hangs onto a blade of grass. It will catch me if I'm not careful and draw me in to exclaim its beauty. Why would I separate out to admire it and be caught? I stand up suddenly and glare up at the heavens then down to Emily on the bank of the river, as if she could rescue me. I see the trap I can't escape. Life gets to live through me; it gets to smell and see and touch this fine flower because of me. I am the body that makes perception, experience, possible. My senses bring a world to life and before I know it I have disappeared, like a leaf in a whirlwind, into the beginningless, endless activity of living.

The music, which was bursting forth like a golden message from on high, tarnishes into monotony. My head is still reverberating from the night of continual noise, underneath the Islamic bombardment.

' Emily, how are you?' My courage is failing.

'I'm fine. Will you check the bread for ants before I put it away? I'll wash the dishes.' She's gentle and perfunctory and squats by the tap with our plates. Should I be embarrassed at how grotty this is? I check the bread and pack it away with our other food. 'Can you help with my pack?' she asks. She must be thinking it's all pretty gross. The toilets are disgusting. What a cheap way of travelling!

On our way to the hosed-out toilets we pass roughly-shaven men hiding behind newspapers on the bench seats. We skirt piles of rubbish left by sweepers. My head is throbbing black and red. I can't jump from unriddling the universe one minute to deciphering Emily's moods the next.

'We've a three-hour bus trip ahead of us. I need something for my head. Maybe coffee will help.'

'There's a coffee bar in the supermarket. Come with me.'

She strides across the dusty street. Stubby regrowth hair and long thick legs grow from her pack. Her smile, when she turns to see if I'm following, is beautiful. I relax.

The instant coffee is super weak. At the small, grey formica table, packs dumped in the corner, Emily restless, I'm reduced to moaning and clutching my head

'This tastes like dishwater.' I trek back to the counter for another teaspoon.

'I'm going to check my email. I'll meet you back here.'

I follow her out with my eyes and look around. The café opens into a bustling supermarket of women floating past in shining saris and embroidered dresses. Young girls, in colourful tops and fitted skirts, gather shyly to chat. The scene is a glittering spectacle of jewellery, patterns, coloured cloth and curled or smooth hair tamed into buns and plaits or falling loose. I dissolve in the flowing cloth curving around slender bodies, limbs graceful, pushing carts, jewelled fingers paying money. I slip inside the voices, the excited gossip, realising how hungry I am for this delicate grace.

'Okay, time to go.' I brace myself for the transition.

'Jack hasn't written.' Emily clumsily picks up her pack.

She walks out. Her face says it all: I have no other life to live and this one is boring and yuck. What else would I be doing? Getting bored somewhere else?

We jostle our heavy packs back across to the market place. We stow them on the bus in overhead racks meant for hand luggage and I worry they might fall. My eyes close. I sink inwards so my curdled brain can soften. After a few minutes, my eyes gently open and stare into the ceaseless agitation, called living, going on outside the bus. The women shop purposefully, the men hang about, ready if an offer of work or conversation should come along. Small dry leaves flitter across the gravel, stirring in bus exhaust then falling to the hot tar seal when the gust moves on. A woman in a bright blue sari is picking through fruit in a barrel, lost in what she's doing.

I gaze around. Everything is extraordinarily present and precious. A roughly-dressed Fijian crosses aimlessly in front of our bus, a rangy dog noses for scraps – they both ooze the glory of existence. Emily's thigh presses solidly against mine. I feel the day-pack, rough and uncomfortable on my lap. I glance across Emily out the window. The bus snorts away from the depot and rumbles through town heading for the jungle.

The road is not the way it looks on our map. The map shows a straight dark line. I thought my spiritual path was a straight dark line, taking me all the way to liberation. Maps are helpful but deceptively over-simplified, I decide. We bounce over gaping potholes and stop to inch through deep mud in treacherous grooves. We follow a silvery snaking river inland – the way I follow fine silvery threads of feeling down into my body when I'm meditating.

'Emily, what do you think? My plastic dinghy could float the two of us down this silvery trail easily. We could camp the nights on the river bank.'

'That would be so much fun.' Emily doesn't take me too seriously. She's not meant to, but she does think it would be cool.

We bump along through dark virgin rainforest. Young men carry heavy sacks of green bananas to the roadside. Young plants sprout in small clearings. A dark woman squats by the road, by her bananas. The faraway look in her eyes startles me. It's like a cross between the intelligence I've seen in a cat's eyes and the eyes of a wise being. I wonder how she thinks.

'Look, Emily, the fence posts are sprouting into trees.'

She's not a child. She doesn't want to be disturbed – she's dreaming about Jack, wondering why he hasn't written, wondering if they're over. She rummages about in the bag to make up for feeling so mean. 'Do you want some food? We have passion fruit, bananas and some crackers.'

I hold out my hand like a grateful child.

The countryside is wild and beautiful. Gentle pasture vanishes into forest and the slow river keeps reappearing. Clothes dry on river stones, bamboo rafts knock against the bank, cassava grows in the gravel left over from making the road and unterraced garden plots trace the hills. Young men appear from the jungle, their eyes wild and unfocused – souls stirred by energies and feelings I can only wonder about. It's humbling to observe from the comfort of the bus. I stare after them. Brown hands and feet, brown bodies, brown soil – children of the land. My heart bursts with longing. I travel like a penniless hobo to return me to her.

The bus drops us at the next town. At the money machine the receipt says: 'no available funds.' Maybe the bank suffered a drought; I wouldn't know this far away. Emily tries her card. When the mechanical shuffle of counting money starts, my sweat dries up. Very little rent is going into my account to cover the large monthly mortgage payments going out.

Another bus drops us in Suva. We will bus into the interior tomorrow. The streets and the shops are reassuringly familiar. Emily is buoyed by the trendy lingerie and home decoration shops. We study another map and lug our heavy packs to the outskirts of town.

'Why can't we get a taxi?' Emily mutters grumpily to herself.

Sweaty dust dripping into our mouths, we climb too many steps and then lean against the large glass doors of a grand colonial hotel-turned-backpackers. A polite Fijian woman appears out of the dark wood and the floral carpet to show us our room. The high ceiling is a shock. The walls are flat blue, without texture, still and quiet. I haven't felt anything as crisp as the white sheets on our beds in years. Emily dances around like she's been rescued from a nightmare, then falls down onto the bed, smiling.

'This is how it's supposed to be,' she declares. 'There'll be white people here, like us, to talk to.'

'I'm going for a shower. I hope the water's hot,' I giggle.

'I'll go after you. I want to look around first.'

She unpacks. I linger under the hot water, directing the pressure onto my tight shoulders and back. I wash my face over and over and splash soap bubbles all over my soft tummy for longer than I should.

Our room-mate, a young Brazilian woman with long brown hair and oily bronze skin, appears in the doorway. She's decorated top to toe in beads and feathers and has been here for months, making jewellery, waiting for her boyfriend. She snips leather and threads beads through the night, keeping me well enough awake to hear the comings and goings from bars and clubs and the bedrooms of other guests, and well enough awake to fret about our plans and about Dad.

In the morning I scrub at my dragging tiredness with a second shower. We breakfast on fried taro and cassava. We need to be ready for anything and eat more than we normally would.

Is it the tiredness? The room starts fading into burning flames of light. Something in me is out of balance.

'Well, Mum, what's the plan?' She hands me a cup of tea.

I drink and think. 'We'll bus into the interior of the island today, walk to where we can camp or stay the night in a village, and then walk through the jungle across to the other side. We'll stay on the road all the way, so we won't get lost, and we should meet up with a bus the other side. How does that sound?'

'Fine. How do we get to stay in a village?'

'I have no idea. I've never stayed in a village. We have a tent, so whatever happens we'll be fine. If there aren't any buses out, we'll hitch. Our adventures have all worked out so far. We're still alive.'

'That's encouraging.' Emily feigns a long groan. 'I wish we hadn't brought so much stuff.'

She is not complaining, just stating the obvious. We packed for any eventuality, except traipsing around on foot for miles. Our packs are ridiculously heavy, crammed with tinned food, body creams in heavy glass containers, snorkelling gear, cooking gear and lots of clothes. We can give the tinned food away.

'I hope the weather gets better. I don't want to be walking in this grey rain.' Emily states the obvious again, almost flippantly, as she tugs the hood over her pack and tightens the straps.

I push my clothes down into all the spaces around the snorkelling gear and jars, so everything will fit.

'Let's stay here in the sunroom. We have two hours before the bus.'

Nothing is certain about our little adventure. The sunroom is stale and unfriendly. Outside, grey cloud gathers and spits of rain hang on the glass.

Emily reads. I fold my legs up on a vinyl wooden-armed chair and worry about Dad. I hope he's made some friends. He's probably happier without us. How disappointed is he in me?

I cross my legs the other way around – the chair's pretty uncomfortable. I could join Emily on the small sofa. Images of Dad – sitting on the boat smoking, stooped, pottering around the engine, walking to the Northerner to look for a drinking partner – float up. I can't save him from his loneliness, but I didn't even try. Dark clouds rolled between us. I don't know where they came from. My mind rushes carelessly on and on, panicky, because I can't get rid of the guilt. The heavy pack I carry on my back has a lot of my father in it.

The small hour hand creeps around the face of my watch until it says we can go. Inner anxiety flips to outer anxiety. The clear glass doors of civilisation close behind as we step down into the unknown. I shiver involuntarily.

'Wow! Another air-conditioned bus.' Emily pretends to be excited.

Air-conditioned in Fiji means no glass. She plays with the loose blinds that unroll to keep out rain and cold. The seats fill up with burly Fijians. The jungle of the interior belongs to them. The rainforest is thick and wet and hard to coax a living from. Indians stay on the plains where they can grow sugar cane and animals.

The bus radio blasts slow, sentimental songs from the sixties, mixed up with local folk music and Fijian news broadcasts. The sound overload knocks my headache out of hiding. Emily disappears into a book, to keep away from me. We're squished in a small two-seater, bodies snuggled together for physical contact only. Progress is slow with the bus stopping frequently at undercover shops. They aren't really that – it's just their walls aren't plastered with coke and cigarette advertising. Dark heavy Fijians clamber down and return with bags and bags of white bread, food, petrol and large cardboard boxes of meat. The aisle piles high.

I match the creeping slowness of the bus, the constant slowing down, stopping, starting up. I follow the disembarking and embarking passengers. I look down into conversations as families come back together and friends depart. The afternoon rumbles slowly along the metal road into the heavy brooding jungle. Great vines threaten the lives of the trees. (They were planted by Americans to provide camouflage for troops and equipment during the war.) Stands of giant bamboo rise up and then soften, feathery tops falling outwards in a big welcome.

My mind sinks. I let it alone. I am too weary to shape it, to even begin to help it soften and open out like the bamboo. Uninvited, tentative, starting slowly from my toes, the threads of a new awareness creep upwards through my body. I start. What is this? I'm like someone who's been in search of a rare bird. I catch a glimpse and I know for sure what it is. This quality of awareness is coming from outside of me. It's from the land. My body rushes with excitement.

I want to shout out: 'Emily, I've found it! I've found it! I can feel it. The consciousness of the land is seeping up through my toes, my legs! Can you feel it? I've found what I have been looking for.'

I do nothing with the bubbling excitement. Emily would think I was crazy. We travel on. Mostly, we're driving through heavy jungle and cold windy rain. Villages appear where jungle has been cleared. I don't know where we're going and it doesn't matter. The land has called me back to her.

Laseleva, lying on the bend of a river, nestles in hills rising up behind. The bus stops and we get down for a break. I can't wait to wriggle my toes in the soil. A woman from the bus offers to take us to a toilet. I realise how cold it is in the bus – the air conditioning is set too low. The land rushes up through my feet, warm and thick – a grounding quality of mind, not body. I stand steady, stable, feet rooted in the land.

The village woman is excited. 'Come, come, over here.'

She leads us proudly through her village to the toilet. My legs walk through the land as if the land belonged to me and I belonged to the land. The feeling is totally natural, the most natural feeling in the world. We were always together – it's just I forgot. I follow Emily back onto the bus. It rumbles on through the rain, into the night, and in the soft light a young woman comes up and introduces herself.

'Hello. My name is Maree. I'm the community nurse at Nagalewai. Would you like to come and stay at my home with my husband and daughter?' Her English is good, her smile bright and welcoming.

'We'd love to stay. Thank you so much. We'll leave early in the morning for Navai.' I don't want to be a burden.

At seven o'clock, after six hours driving through jungle, we arrive. Emily is finally impressed. Mum came through with a place to stay in the dismal jungle.

14

We follow Maree and her family through the partially-fenced garden. The front door opens into the living room, where a picture of Jesus smiles down. The room is bare except for a TV, VCR, stack of videos in one corner and one chair. Mali, the husband, puts on a video and collapses into the chair. The house has two fluorescent lights, one in the living room and one in the kitchen. I drop my pack against a wall and follow Maree into the kitchen.

'Is this all you have to cook on?' I try to keep my voice even, staring at a single- element kerosene stove.

'Yes. I heat all our water and cook all our meals here. I must apologize. We don't have running water at the moment. Something has broken.'

'I'm used to camping and living on a boat. Life is very simple there too, so don't worry.'

The house is musty and dirty, the walls and ceiling grey with mould.

'My daughter's room has a bed and a settee. You can sleep there.'

'Where will she sleep?'

'She can sleep with us. I'm sorry the house is so untidy. I've been away all week at another village. Their nurse was sick.'

She picks up a grass broom and starts sweeping.

I smile, 'Your home is lovely. I'm the same when people arrive unexpectedly at my place – I start sweeping. I'd love a cup of tea.' That's an understatement. 'Six hours in a bus is a long time for me without tea.' She puts water on the stove and we sit on the floor of her daughter's bedroom for some white bread and butter. 'I've got Orere quince jelly in my pack.'

Maree passes jellied bread to Mali and her daughter.

'Living here in the village is so difficult, we have no money and we can't do anything. I barely earn enough to support my family. I want to go to England and nurse. My brother works there.'

'What do you do?' I ask Mali.

'I look after the house while Maree works.' He smiles weakly. 'Once a week I go back to my village. I have land there.'

'What do you grow?'

'Kava, taro and cassava.'

'I want to tell you about my life,' Maree interrupts. 'I was very unhappy as a teenager, I was all alone and angry. I took lots of drugs and got pregnant. I felt so worthless and useless, I wanted to die. Then I found God and my life completely changed. Now it makes sense. Jesus is my friend. I'm never alone because he's always there. I know what love is. I trained as a nurse, so I can help others.' She pauses to butter another slice of bread. 'You're the first white people I've had in my home.'

A loud scuffling in the hallway interrupts us. Two people burst into the room, flushed with excitement. Maree recognises them, so I relax.

'A man from Mali's village has cut himself. He's bleeding badly. We need to go now to help him. Can you and Mali come with us?'

Maree explains: 'They're nurses from a nearby village. The message must have come by radio. They need Mali to show the way to his village. At night we travel in large groups for safety.'

I stare at her mouth, following the shaping of the words, and up to her bright eyes and her dark curly hair. I can't believe our luck – we have an adventure into the interior, just like that!

'Can we come with you?' I won't accept no. I'll plead and beg if I have to. I won't stay behind.

'We have to walk several hours upstream in the dark. It's the only way to get there – there's no road.' She looks doubtful.

We'd be walking into the very heart of Fiji. My heart leaps. 'We'd love to come.'

I look across to Emily. She smiles under the pressure of my urgent glance. Doesn't she realise what an adventure this is, how lucky we are? Her face doesn't light up. She doesn't want to miss out and stay here all by herself, but it does seem like a lot of hard work. She'd rather play with Liu, the six-year-old daughter.

Maree's as excited as me and looks at Emily encouragingly. 'Of course you can come.'

She takes Liu to a friend's house. I fill our daypack with snacks, torches and warm thermal tops. My excitement refuses to acknowledge my extreme tiredness. My headache is worse. At eleven o'clock, when we close the front door and set out into the dark night, it's hammering solidly. I swallow another couple of Panadol.

Behind town we follow the bank straight down into the river. I don't think about eels or water monsters – I have worse problems. My leather sandals stretch in the water and my feet start sliding all over the place. I don't want to take them off; barefoot may be worse.

'I can't stand on slippery rocks. I'm not usually like this,' I apologise. 'It's my sandals.'

Mali reaches out to help. There are twenty-four river crossings to come. My mind stretches like my sandals, until it's deep under the water and rocks, where my sandals would slide me without Mali's help. We push across the strong current, often waist or chest high, through the bubbling turbulence sweeping us around.

Emily wades ahead and strides out onto the far bank. Her headlamp wobbles over the rocks. Maree is only just keeping up. The other couple are in the middle. I lose sight of Emily when she disappears down into the next crossing. I love it all. I'm sure Mali enjoys helping the weak white woman I've become, as much as I enjoy depending on his strength. He rushes into the forest and returns with large bamboo poles, then proceeds to smash the ends with a rock until they're fibrous. They become fiery torches, dancing flames, bright and warm, but they slow us down. We have to continually relight the glowing charcoal from other torches that are still bright.

Behind my searing headache, I look out from an unfamiliar blank darkness. The earth has taken me away to her domain. My head is like the shell of a burnt-out house. Stumbling along with my fire-torch, I follow Mali, broken to pieces inside. I can't gather myself together as a whole solid ball of me, self-contained and safe, nor can my sandals.

We walk along a muddy track, across stony river flats and plunge again and again into the dark river, following the torches, which break into smaller groups and then come back together in different ways, like the refrain of a simple tune.

'The rain hasn't stopped for over a week,' Mali tells me. 'That's why the river is so high.'

The sky is overcast, starless and moonless. The shadowy dancing light of bamboo torches brings the surrounding rock to life. I see scrub on its way to forest, white water breaking over stones. I can barely see in front of my feet most of the time. I twice fall into the white foam, the broken water like my mind, stumbling over dark shadows. I don't get cold even though I'm wearing a thin silk shirt and shorts.

'We'll stop to rest here,' Mali commands as the leader. We come together under an arching rock, the way a small clan of hunter-gatherers might, crouching close together, absorbed into the dark shadow. I share around bread and bananas from my pack. Mali relights the fading torches and we set off again, into the night, heading towards morning.

He rushes ahead and then returns, smiling broadly. 'We're here!'

I look up perplexed. I don't understand. I forgot our walking would come to an end. My watch tells me we set out four and a half hours ago. It's 3:30 am. After clambering up the muddy bank and across soft wet grass, we head for a simple corrugated iron hut – the nurses' station in this isolated village of Lasoga.

I immediately curl up under a blanket, on my third of the bed. Emily lies down next to me and we fade into oblivion. The patient with the gashed leg arrives soon after. The whole village comes down to see us sleeping; they want to wake us up and share tea, but Maree stops them.

'You're the first white people ever to arrive here in the night,' Maree says brightly next morning.

I turn to Emily, 'Well, here we are, in the heart of Fiji, with real jungle people.'

This is not her dream come true. 'Yes, we're here. I need some dry clothes.' She looks around. 'Where's the toilet?' She stretches and yawns. 'I'm going to see.'

The house is surrounded by sloshy mud. The toilet is outside. Rusting corrugated iron huts, like this one, scatter over the hillside and beyond. Muddy tracks snake through the grass, joining them.

'It rains every day.' Maree hands me a bundle of dry clothes. 'They belong to the nurse who's usually here, but she's on leave at the moment. She won't mind you wearing them.'

I poke around the different rooms: bedroom, clinic rooms, kitchen/living room. I guess the brightly-coloured wall posters come from New Zealand. They explain concepts of self respect and patient rights, and how counselling can help.

'Come, come, they're waiting for us. It's time to go,' Maree urges. 'Mali's sister, Gina, has cooked us breakfast.'

We trudge barefoot through the rain and wash our muddy feet at the entrance. About thirty people, mainly women, are sitting on the floor, waiting. Bowls of food steam and cool on a long white cloth laid over woven floor mats. Pretty ornaments, pictures and flowers decorate the room. Beaten cloth hangs from the walls. The simple blend of formality and homeliness surprises me – it contrasts so sharply with everything about our sailing trip. We don't have any formality on our boat, or homeliness; I don't do either very well. The art of civilisation has been finely-tuned here. Everything means something; the ornaments have a history. Children touch them, grown-ups tell their story. Someone here made the woven mats and beaten cloth. This room is the pride of these people – it hums with light and family ties.

We eat boiled cassava, pancake, yam, meat stew and sip tea from large bowls. Gina is a warm and gracious host. I forget the mud and rain outside.

After the meal, the male ritual of drinking kava starts. Dark hands squeeze water through a cheesecloth full of powdered kava, into a bowl. They pour the elixir into a half coconut shell and, clapping, offer it around the circle of men, one person at a time. This kava ritual is what the men do when they're not working. I try a couple of bowls. The effect, apart from sharpening my headache, is extremely pleasant. A soft contentment washes through me.

Emily tunes a loosely-strung guitar and sings wistfully to its accompaniment. We sing, in harmony, the song we've always sung together, on long car trips and around campfires: New Zealand's real national anthem, Pokarekare Ana. I'm always moved by its beauty, no matter how badly or how often we sing it. Our contribution made, Emily passes the guitar into the circle of men. I sink down into the thick nest of dried grass under the matting; I don't want to ever get up.

After a few hours of sleep back at our hut, Maree calls us awake, and we traipse back through rain and mud to share dinner with the whole village this time. We sit with the women in front of boiled yam, cassava, taro and meat. The men sit and stand behind us, and eat after we have finished.

The women speak very little English. I challenge the shy smiles of the children. 'What's your name?' They show me things, then rush away, watch, get brave with a question and dissolve into soundless giggles. I wish I could talk with the women, but my head's not working well, I can't think clearly. This much is all I can do.

My mind is deep in the earth, growing dark soil into thick rough tubers far from the sun. Taro and cassava are the staple of every meal here. Every footstep carries mud. The village is isolated from the outside world by impassive, brooding rainforest on all sides. Grey sullen rain falls every day. The abiding atmosphere in the room is heavy and resigned rather than contented and creative. Money from kava and other crops is traded for salt, kerosene and flour. I ask a young kava-drinking man about education.

'Most teenagers go to high school in Suva. They board with relatives. The boys usually come back to the village when they finish, but the girls don't. They go into further training or find work in town.' He talks easily, his English is good, but he looks unhappy. 'I came back to the village after high school. Now I want to leave. I hate it here – I have no life, but I have no training and no money.' He takes another bowl of kava. 'I don't know how to get away.'

The men have kava, the women have each other and their children. The women are yeast in a heavy mix. The sweetness and warmth in their voices lifts the night from an otherwise heavy monotony.

Early next morning, Gina arrives to say goodbye, bringing pancakes, slices of pawpaw and tea. She waves us down the grassy slope to the river. I'm embarrassed that I don't have a gift for her. My headache has softly faded, so we all set out in good spirits down the river. I'm ready to play! I don't need sandals, I can see the rocks and leap confidently from plateau to plateau, that is until my little toe crashes into a stubborn stone. 'Damn it.'

'What is it, Mum?'

'My toe, I think it's broken. I can't put any weight on it. Just when I was okay again. I can't believe it! ' I walk on slowly.

'Do you want one of my soft boat shoes?'

'No, I'm fine. I'll be okay.' I have to pay attention to every step, weighting my foot with no pressure on my little toe, placing the ball very softly on each stone. An hour of this is long enough. 'It's too sore. Emily, can I have a shoe after all?'

'Of course. Are you okay?' We walk together a while and chat. 'It's strange, Mum. Maree is so friendly and nice and yet I feel dissatisfied all the time. What upsets me is that I can't think of anything I could do, with anyone, anywhere, that would make me happy.' I smile, pleased for once to have a reply: 'It's not things that make you happy. Real happiness is something you bring to the circumstances of your life, not something you find in life.'

'Do you think so?'

'Of course. We are naturally happy – look at children.'

Emily slows down, curious and irritated by my confidence. She's sick to death of her moods, they're destroying her holiday.

'Sometimes I am happy,' Emily ponders, 'but it doesn't stay.'

'I know, I'm the same. For some reason we're determined to cling to our yukky states.'

Emily looks slightly embarrassed; she knows what I'm saying is true. When she starts to let go she panics, like she's about to disappear with her mood, so she picks it up again.

We wade into the water, struggling again to stay upright against the flow.

'Let's swim. It'll be fun and easier on your toe,' Emily suggests.

The others follow us in, laughing as the bubbling water floats us way downstream to our far bank. Chocolate and biscuits from my day pack feed us all. The return journey has taken a little over three hours. It's Sunday – church music entangled in mist sanctifies the village.

Maree goes straight to work at the nurse's station next door, offering medicines and advice to a trickle of women and children. Emily and I get to be alone, resting on the front veranda, two large cups of strong coffee for me. The sun sends shards of light through holes in the churning grey cloud.

'You know, Mum, what you were saying about happiness – you're right. The problem's inside me.' She drifts happily back to her book.

I'm left musing about my romance with the land. I think back to Bible stories, myths and fables, stories of exile and return. I keep missing the land. I want to return, but not back to village life. I would be like the young kava-drinking man, and Maree, hell bent on my freedom. So what is this deal I have about the land? What on earth am I on about when I say I want to wake the land up in me, that I want to know myself as the land? I feel slightly embarrassed and yet I can't escape the power of the earth. What is real and what is fantasy?

Emily and I stay on the front porch, writing and reading, catching sunlight when it falls our way. A woman from across the road sees us alone.

'Hello,' she says confidently, in very good English.

I look up and suddenly feel like I'm meeting an old friend.

'My name is Jeanine. You haven't been welcomed to this village. I know you've been away. Will you come to my house and drink kava?'

Her face is proud and thoughtful.

'Of course.' I turn to Emily – she doesn't look pleased. 'Come on, Emily.'

Jeanine's father is an important member of the village and the house is large and clean with closed verandahs and polished floors. We sit against the wall of a large empty room. The men sit cross-legged in the centre, clapping and offering the half-coconut bowl of muddy kava. No one says much. This is about as dull as an afternoon could possibly get. I'm not much good with dull. Children sneak in around us.

'Jeanine, why don't we go play some games with the children?'

She's too polite not to agree. 'Of course, if you'd like to.'

I teach them 'Simon says do THIS', with star jumps and touching toes and then 'Simon says do THAT,' to get them out. Emily jumps up and collects stones from outside to play knuckle bones.

'We'll do a skit,' I coax Emily.

Emily sits in a chair and takes her arms out of her T-shirt. I crouch down behind and put my arms through the sleeves to replace her arms. She acts out a teenage girl getting ready for her first date. The children laugh and laugh as I clumsily comb her hair and spread lipstick over her face with her substitute hands. Then we laugh as they proudly act out stories they learned at school. Am I surprised to discover they are as talented and precocious as my children were at their age?

Jeanine and I leave the children with Emily and sit in front of the kettle boiling over a warm fire. She seems content and fulfilled as a mother. I remember the feeling. I could stay all evening, I have so many questions.

'Do Fijians marry for love?' I ask.

She smiles. 'My husband-to-be went to my father with a whale's tooth. It was an offer too good to refuse.'

I wonder if Fijian women are as preoccupied with their relationships as we are in the west. What could she say to Emily about romance? I don't have a chance to ask, and what could she say? The children gather around and we all sing together. Her pure voice carries strongly above us. Something inside her is all alone. The children are getting tired and grizzly – time to go.

We've been gone too long and return to an anxious household. Maree didn't know where we were and is worried. Maybe not worried – maybe she thought we belonged to her and is put out that we went next door. I don't know and it doesn't matter. I chat extra-enthusiastically while she cooks pancakes. I'm used to this. The carrier leaves at half past four in the morning and Mali has booked our seats. I tie a large flax mat woven by Mali's sister onto my pack and, in the front pocket, store some freshly-fried taro for breakfast. We exchange addresses and promise letters. They are sad to see us go so soon and we are grateful for their warm hospitality.

15

The road is in such an appalling state, the buses won't use it anymore. Our carrier, a small truck with a six-by-two plank to sit on and a thin iron rod to lean back against, bumps over the heavily-pitted road. We are squashed up against children and adults to make room for great wands of kava root, scent from the long colourfully tied stems soothing the dark cold night. Mist hangs heavy in the valleys, moon and stars peep from sweeping cloud. Rumbling towards dawn, away from the dark interior into gentle grassy slopes, I wake slowly from my dream of tangled, untamed wildness and sullen dark men. We rumble to the east coast: concrete paths, painted houses, pretty gardens, women in silky brocades and boxer-shorted children. The carrier unloads at Tavua, north of Lautoka.

'I'm going to find a café,' Emily grumps. Sometimes she breaks free, most of the time she doesn't. Maybe it's to do with me. I'm like this with Dad, so I have to deal with myself in her. That's karmic justice!

Jack still hasn't written. She's trying to stay objective, to just observe, but she can't. We shop, with me hobbling because my painful toe won't take any weight. Lugging packs, bags of food and the large woven mat, we catch a bus to Raviravi, two hours north, the place we stayed our first night out. From there a taxi to Ellington wharf, where an open boat ferries us out to a small island, Na-nui-ra.

Tent pitched, I put on the kettle for tea and slip, just like that, into a totally different circumstance. It hasn't rained here for weeks and the ground is dry and hard. A cool wind rustles dry coconut fronds and teases the sea, reminding me of Oliver teasing the irresistible Charlotte when they were children. Lying on our woven mat under

coconut palms, not directly under the young green coconuts though
– they can kill you with a direct hit – our faces brush dry airy space.
We relax, no longer a curiosity in someone else's life. Waves crash
onshore, cattle graze the pasture over the fence and I stroll around,
as fresh and light as the breeze flapping my clothes dry.

A boatload of 'Fijian Experience' youngsters arrive. They fill the
empty tents and dorms with forced excitement, moving awkwardly
between strangers and new friends. Dry wind and sand absorb the
chatter; relentless heat fades them into the background. The loud
portable cassette player on an umbrella table outside revs up the
holiday spirit but, actually, the whole place is dry and empty.

Men are working well into the night on a large building project.
The new kiwi owner confides that she's almost had enough of the two
groups fighting. We hardly notice as we walk around identifying the
different buildings. The kitchen is a jerry-built outhouse with a freezer
for a fridge and brackish water trickling from the taps. Emily drinks
a glass because no one told her not to and vomits and shits through
the night. By morning she's weak and empty – not a good empty. She
starts the day in her usual bog of dissatisfaction. She's bored. We
talk of how to be content with a burning discontent, Krishnamurti
style. When nothing steers the day in an interesting way, we wonder
whether it's possible to live well by just paying attention.

'I don't think attention is enough. Desire kindles the flame of life
– the stronger and clearer our desire, the brighter the flame. I know
spiritual teachers talk about cultivating unconditional, non-clinging
awareness. It may be necessary, but it's not sufficient.'

'I know,' Emily answers. She looks miserable and courageous at
the same time. 'I don't know what I want and I can't pretend I do.'

'Well, I always have a question,' I answer brightly. 'Without a
question I'd feel as lost as you do.' I pass her some cool, boiled water.
'The known is a terribly claustrophobic place to live.'

We laugh for a bit, remembering our time in Lautoka and face into
the afternoon sun with its shadows creeping towards us.

Emily springs up, hollow tummy yawning from under her singlet.
'I need to do some washing.'

I stroll out along the beach with my endless thoughts for company. Wavelets froth on the edge of the shore, a seagull arcs across the sky, the wind rustles around us.

Up in the hills in the cool evening, I stop in the long grass. Emily walks on. My aching toe makes walking difficult. Sometimes I wonder if my questioning will ever come to an end, if I will ever give up the hook for a full stop. I gaze into space and follow an old niggle. I spent years studying different theories on truth. At university, truth was related to statements. A statement was true if it fit the facts and false if it didn't. Just what a fact was, was more of a problem than the philosophers had a ready answer for. I'm sure 'truth' is about something quite different. Philosophers keep well away from this different kind of 'truth'. They hold up bunches of garlic. When Jesus said, 'I am the way, the truth and the life,' he wasn't talking about true statements.

I gaze out over the frisky water. I've seen truth, in the glorious present moment. I've tracked it down, but it never stays.

At dusk, half past five, Emily and I sit in brightly-painted Cape Cod chairs on the golden sand, bathed now in the setting sun. Evening falls and a cool onshore breeze wriggles through openings in my fisherman pants and singlet. I leave to make dinner, bare feet pricking on the spiky grass. Washing out a pot to cook up a tuna pasta has the feeling of forever going nowhere about it, an ambiance of space and light.

We slip into a soft sofa in the communal lounge, with cups of tea. It's empty but for the painter of murals, a well-travelled man, painting the concrete block and wooden buildings here into thatch, grand seascapes and floral, butterfly-filled jungle. He definitely has a gift. They look great, not kitschy and cheap, but flamboyant and fun. He's eccentric and about my age – eccentric because somewhere he got lost in his own grand exposition of life. He doesn't want to hear our stories, only to delight in his own, through us, to keep himself alive. He brings out a photo album of murals he painted all over the world.

He looks at Emily. When I ask questions, he answers her open smile.

'I was in Kashmir, doing nothing in particular, waiting, eating bean sprouts and stuff.' His words slur only slightly. He's a wiry, tanned Kiwi who, like Dad and me, took on the radical task of the sixties and seventies – reclaiming life from the city dump of social expectation and control. We wrestled free of social responsibility into a crisis of identity that propelled us with great speed at different bullseyes: freedom, adventure, spirituality, new age ideas, drugs, love.

The painter of murals is earnest and confiding: 'I didn't know where I was going. I meditated a little, looked at the voices in my head, sorted out where I came from, made friends with my issues.' He makes a sideways comment to the lady manager about using herbs instead of Viagra. 'One day I started painting. I was never into drawing or painting as a child, nothing like that. I became a colour therapist. I started channelling colour and now my work has taken me all over the world.'

Emily looks at him. He turns to her. 'You're a very spiritual person and one day you will know your purpose. You have nothing to worry about.' He opens a page in his photo album and we gather close to admire the magnificent murals. He turns the page as if he's turned it too many times. Under the friendly exposition I sense an ennui, maybe he's the half-baked fallout of a hippy movement that flew too high on drugs and sex. I can recognise fallout – I'm the fallout of too much exciting spiritual experience. He seems to have made a good life for himself. I've always been suspicious of people like him, who have a ready answer for everything, but I'm also drawn to their easy ways.

Emily looks from him to me as if to ask: 'Am I meant to take him seriously? Is he Mercury carrying a message from the gods or a drunken old hippy away with the fairies?'

I smile back an implicit encouragement. I want to believe in him.

The next morning she confides: 'Mum, I'm happier today. I was okay with being unhappy, though.'

I turn from the dishes I'm washing in the grubby kitchen. 'What did you think of the painter of murals? He said something special to you.'

Emily sits down at a sloppily-painted table and picks up the coconut scraper. The worker here gave us coconuts and we're following her directions, scraping the white meat with the metal fingers, and squeezing the shreds through cheesecloth to extract the milk.

'I feel reassured by what he said. Maybe that's why I'm happy today.'

The board under her scraper fills with a second pile of fluffy white flesh.

My arms, bubbly with detergent, swing the air. 'I'm sure all is as it should be. You aren't meant to be pursuing the known, you're waiting for the unknown to come knocking.'

'Maybe.'

We dip our fingers into the bowl of fresh coconut cream, and dribble it down our chins.

Each day we venture a little further over the island and the next day walk up over the ridge and down to a long ribbon of golden sand on the far side. Glossy-leafed branches reach out over sand, as far from their roots as they dare. It's quiet except for water lapping the sand. We lie naked in leafy shadow, caressed by the cool onshore breeze. I swim way out to cool off and look for tropical fish, but lose my direction on the way back. How is that possible? I can't see Emily, so I set off up and down the beach in the glorious afternoon sun to find her, further each time until she's there, covered in shining sparkles of sand.

Suddenly it is all too beautiful, too beautiful to stand. It's as if my mind can't stand the intensity, the hugeness of this actual life, and so it escapes, it flies off out into space all around, and then it turns around and looks directly back into my life, a shocking sight. It can see who I am, all the performances, all the strategies, all the faces I take on, spinning me round and round without knowing. It sees my human story and I feel finished with it all, not interested. Sadness seesawing with happiness, loneliness plugging anger, enthusiasm covering emptiness? I'm done. Let me out. I don't want any names in this great cauldron of life. I don't want to curdle out. I want to stay here behind and beyond all my births. Please let me stay. I'm aching all over to stay rescued. I can't stand what I'm seeing. It's not okay.

I wrap a crimson sarong around my naked skin and set out for home, walking into the setting sun. My body walks without me. The ocean is as still as the breathless, cloudless sky – shimmering sea, hills, scrubby plants, browsing cattle – all arising from the vast womb of nothing. We walk through a track under arching trees. Emily strides way out in front. The niggle comes back. It's always the same. I know this place – it's not a human place. It's not where people eat and make love. It doesn't have toes wriggling in sand. I can't stay. I don't know where to make my home.

I let Emily go further ahead. I break twigs off a tree and scrunch them to pieces in my hand. I stop as if I have the choice not to walk any further. I don't. I don't want to keep walking, caught in this blind repetitive game. I put one foot in front of the next. I can't change the way it is. I have to stride up the hill. I don't get to make the rules of the game.

I sit in long silky grass and watch the sun slip away, its work done. The luminous shining disc throws beams of golden-orange light. Where does it get the courage to be so dramatic on its way to the sea? Is it free or is it caught in the game?

The boat is some way away. Our packs are ready. Emily has a balancing act for us. She lies on the hard ground, lower legs vertical, feet on my buttocks. I lift up and lean back against her legs while she straightens them. I keep arching backwards until her hands support my shoulders and then I pull against her calves and raise myself into a shoulder stand on her hands. As if that wasn't a triumph enough, she tells me to fold forwards into the plough posture, in the air over her. Her feet move around to support my thighs and she releases her hands.

'This is so, so cool! This is what we get to do in the world to make living worthwhile.' The words come out a little strained as my chin is scrunched into the my chest. After tumbling to the ground, I want more, straight away. 'Can I get up on your shoulders – for old time's sake?' I climb up like a monkey while she leans forward, until I'm sitting, then squatting, then standing on her shoulders. The bitter-sweet of life takes me by surprise. I let go her hands and brace my ankles against her neck. Intense pleasure explodes through me. Pride and glee and pure exhilaration are followed by the stabbing pain of knowing I won't get to do this much more – I'm getting old and life is rushing me on. She walks a tentative few steps, then raises her hands for me. I want this to go on and on, I love it. I climb down her bony back and jump back to the ground. Some days I see through the game, other days I will give anything to play it.

16

The bus drops us near the Vuda Point marina, under the large mango tree bearing its weight of unripe fruit. They are destined to ripen. I gather up some windfall.

We lift the weight of each other's packs and wriggle-force our arms under the straps. Blood rushes to our hot thighs pounding the gravel back to the marina, past the office, past taxis drivers resting against shaded car bonnets and onto the concrete rim where *Dream-maker* is tied up. Unwashed, unkempt, dusty and tired, we clamber over lifelines onto the deck.

'Hi, Dad, are you there? We're back,' I call. We've been away nine days.

I don't see the man in the red boat next door watching our arrival with interest.

Dad climbs up into the cockpit, well pleased to see us.

'Hello there,' he hails. 'The intrepid explorers have returned. Come on down and tell me all about your travels. I'll put on the kettle.'

We drop our packs in the cockpit and follow him down. I look around to see what's different and what's the same. Over a cup of tea and coconut biscuits, our travels unravel.

'How've you been?'

'I've been fine. I like being at a marina with people to talk to.' He smiles a little sheepishly. 'Actually, I've put an ad in the paper for a lady companion.'

I nod. 'That's great. I'm glad you had some company. First things first – we need a shower. I hope the water's warm.'

Emily grabs the soap, I grab shampoo and fresh towels. Stripped naked, we compare bodies in front of the mirror. Emily's body is like a new plastic doll, smooth, almost doughy. Mine looks carved from knotty wood that was hardened in a fire.

She looks at my reflection as if it belongs to her. Her life grew inside and all around this wiry frame, as a single exploding cell to a desirous babe suckling overflowing breasts. She slept with its arms around her, and bounced for miles in soft front and back backs strapped against its pounding heart.

'Your body looks good, Mum.'

Next morning this body splays out in the cockpit, under the shady dodger – a lifeless ragdoll.

'Who do those legs belong to?' A booming, west-coast American accent disrupts my sloppy dreaming.

I sit up, curious of course, as a big smiling sailor on the boat next to us, looms into view.

'I saw you arrive yesterday. I made friends with your father while you were away. He's quite a man. I hope I'm like him at his age.'

I enjoy his forwardness, and smile. Oops! I've seen him before, in a meditation. I knew we were destined to meet. He looks older, that's all. We chat casually, then turn away and turn back, pulled it seems by hidden strings.

'When did you arrive at Vuda Point?' I ask.

'How long will you be here?' he wants to know. His deep, melodious voice reverberates between our boats.

'Alice, we're about to go into town,' Dad calls up.

'I must go now.' I'm overexcited. He disappears.

Two minutes on shore and I've changed my mind. I'm tired, I'll stay behind.

'Okay, we'll manage.'

Emily's not pleased, but Jack may have written so she has to go.

I give her the shopping list and money, for market fruit and vegetables, then walk around the marina, behind sunglasses and a hat. At the far end, away from morning boat activity, in the quiet shade of a coconut palm, I stare vacantly into the entrance channel.

In *The Little Prince*, Saint Exupery warned me: a dangerous baobab tree grows from a small seed. Unchecked, it can break a planet to pieces. He was careful to weed his planet – he knew the danger. How do I recognize a weed from a beautiful rose? I laugh treacherously. Is a love affair a dangerous weed or a beautiful rose? The Buddha spent fifty years roaming India teaching only one thing: how to recognise weeds and pull them out and how to recognise roses and help them grow.

Monday is half-price pizza night at the resort next to the marina, an enticement to 'live on a shoestring' yachties. I invite Cornelius, cockpit to cockpit, when he re-appears on our third day back.

'Sure, what time do you want to go?'

Dad and Cornelius talk boat stuff; Emily and I giggle nervously as we pass through the large iron gate, guarded by a big, white-shirted smiling Fijian.

'Bula,' we rejoice. I almost skip as we pass the swaying grasses and low lights. The concrete path leads into an open, thatched restaurant with tables and couples and bottles of wine. Waiters and glamorous hostesses brush past, smiling. This is as romantic a picture as could possibly be. Luxuriant palms brush away the last threads of reality.

Cornelius sits at the head of a large table. He's intelligent and articulate. I sit next to him and the rest of the yachting world filters down the polished table.

'Do you like sailing?' he politely enquires.

'I love sailing. I want to sail all around the world.'

'I've sailed around the world. It took six years. I would do it again. Maybe we could sail together?'

My heart somersaults twice. I bite pizza to settle down. Say it again! Is this possible? You would sail around the world with me?

'What did you do before you went sailing?' I ask and sip wine. Do I look better in profile or front on? I can't remember. I've become a silly teenager, giggling and blushing inside. Emily hates it when I get like this.

'I was a Hollywood producer, but the life didn't suit me, it was too ruthless. I couldn't wait to leave. Sailing was my escape. I've been sailing for twenty years now. *Fantasie* is my home.' His eyes smile, his confidence intrigues me. 'Where would you like to sail to first?' he asks. 'I still haven't sailed to the Mediterranean. We could stop in South America on the way. Brazil is a wonderful place for sailors.'

He seems to be as desperate as I am.

'The Med would be fine by me,' I laugh.

I'm not joking. We are sailing over the horizon together in an adventure that justifies leaving everyone behind. I turn to Emily to break the intensity. We order another round of drinks. Emily watches the silliness. She doesn't like it – she doesn't like being pushed aside. She calls me to her and we both end up in nervous giggles.

When we leave, she picks me up off the ground. 'I'm going to carry you back home, Mum.' I snuggle into her arms and calm down, legs hanging loose.

Next morning Emily announces: 'Mum, Cornelius brought this over while you were in the shower.'

Famous Women Before Ten is a coffee-table book full of black and white photos and interviews with Hollywood stars, of all ages, in the morning before the makeup and glamorous clothes go on. I put the book down without really looking. I'm not fascinated with Hollywood – it's not what I'm on about. I'm not interested in fantasy.

'Thanks for the book.' I return it next morning, with a dismissive disregard.

'The photos were taken by the mother of a young sailing friend. It was my way of saying you are beautiful,' he tells me later, when I ask him what he meant by it all.

First time on his boat I peek around for clues. Is this a new adventure? I want to see quality and finesse. Not sure what I'm looking for. Dark varnished mahogany floor, walls and table. That's good? The dark-green striped squabs are good quality? I'm interested. Everything seems clean and well cared for. It classy.

'She's a forty-foot racing sloop-turned-cutter,' he remarks, raising his head slightly in the open space of the companionway.

'What's a cutter?'

'A cutter has two jibs, a sloop only has one. I rigged a second smaller foresail in front of the main jib.' He takes two stainless mugs from slotted homes in the galley. 'I use it all the time, especially for sailing to windward. You can't get a decent aerofoil on a half-rolled jib.' The espresso machine bubbles energetically on the stove. 'Do you take milk and sugar?' His voice is clear and bold, his head bends slightly to miss the ceiling. He's a big man for a small galley.

I nod. In my mind's eye I can see the badly-rolled jib on Dad's boat, all the way to Fiji.

The open layout is the same as on *Dream-maker*, except there aren't cupboards under side portholes in the saloon. No portholes at all, and the flat decks behind the settee, vacated bunks of racing crew long past, pile up with tidily sorted bundles of stuff. The head is open to the front berth. The boat feels empty and lonely. It could be my imagination. The messiness on our boat is comfortable. Framed adventures peer from the walls, tropical fish, glorious islands. No people. He shows me a photo of his old sailing cat. She was lost overboard. We sit side by side with our coffee and talk earnestly about all sorts of things.

'Can I see your passport?'

He says he's 61, but he looks older to me. I do the critical part now, before its too late and my brain has turned to mush. The little hair he has left is white, his facial skin hangs like pastry, his arms are loose and soft and his legs don't look strong. He's big and a little overweight, his upper chest tight and large, from a lifetime of winching in sails I expect. He doesn't get enough exercise, I can tell.

He explains: 'I was six months in Aspen Colorado just before now, watching runway fashion models on cable TV. I didn't have anything else to do.'

I jump up. 'I've enjoyed talking, but I must go. Dad and Emily are waiting and we'll miss the bus if I don't go now.' I put our thermos-sleeved steel cups in the sink. 'Thanks for the coffee.'

'Why don't you all come over for dinner tonight.' He follows me into the galley as if to keep me there. 'I cook a famous chicken stew. A friend sent the pink peppercorns it needs.'

He takes a packet down from behind some plastic containers.

'Pink peppercorns! How exotic. I've never heard of such a thing.' I turn the packet over and over, to savour the moment. 'Sure, we'd love to come. I'll bring some New Zealand wine.'

I have no idea how to sort all this information. The underneath part of me is interested; he has power, confidence, and a dark side.

Shaun, a young Chinese sailor, Emily and Dad sit one side of the table, Cornelius and I, the other. Cornelius dishes up rice and stew; I pour the wine. Neither Emily nor I get much of a chance to talk.

'I helped Shaun buy his first boat,' Cornelius starts out. 'He's determined to be the first Chinese person to sail around the world single-handed.'

Shaun nods and looks embarrassed and grateful. I wonder what he would be like as a lover now my mind is turning over the idea. I pick at the stew, wondering what is so famous about it. Emily and I look at each other with a 'this is pretty ordinary' look. Dad swallows two glasses of wine and launches into conversation. He's entertaining and unstoppable. I get a headache. Cornelius and I don't have even one small chat.

'Come on, Dad, it's time to go home,' I finally interrupt. 'Nice to meet you, Shaun.'

We shake hands again. I linger to let everyone out. Cornelius puts his arms around me, to say goodnight. I'm sure!

I fall asleep smiling all through – I have a male admirer, I'm back in the game.

Emily and I sit out in the cockpit and talk through the morning to patch up the intrusion of this new man. Inside me is spinning out of control, mincing my guts into a kind of vacant long drop.

'The chicken stew, what was that all about?' we laugh.

I need to be distracted from a debilitating, out of control feeling. I return to the rational me, the part that evaluates carefully, and considers. I try to explain to Emily the ideas that drive me, the serious nature of my questing, so that I can still believe in it. I reawaken the mystery of the nature of perception, the mystery we're embedded in. 'It's clear to me that matter arises in mind rather than the other way around.'

Emily hardly reacts. She's not sure whether to listen properly or to wait silently until I run out of steam. She's happy for us to just be here together out in the sun.

'Perception is a mental phenomenon ... ' This game is leading nowhere. 'Don't you want to understand yourself and life? Aren't you curious about 'truth'?'

'To be honest, Mum, sometimes I think you use 'spirituality' as a way of not dealing with ordinary life. What does it matter to me if space is mind or matter? Mind and matter – maybe they're different words for the same thing.'

I start to answer and then stop; I don't need to argue with her.

Emily stirs uncomfortably. I imagine she's remembering the past, that I've triggered a recurring resentment, something we've never properly faced.

'You've never forgiven me for going away on meditation retreats when you were young.'

Emily turns to me with a hard face. 'It was worse for Charlotte, she was much younger.'

'When you were young, I had no idea what love was. When I turned the word over, nothing happened – the word hung in empty space. Somewhere deep inside I knew that without love nothing mattered at all. My spiritual journey has been about finding love.'

I need to diffuse a sense of debilitating inadequacy and the affront of having to justify my life. I'm not that confident.

'Your life has been hard, but it would have been much harder if I had remained a conventional, angry and unreal mum.'

I start to shake from all my wounds, bruising against imagined walls of resistance. 'No one realises the progress I've made.'

'Mum, it's okay. I love you. Don't get so upset. I do understand what you've done and I admire you for it.'

'Thank you.' I give her a warm hug. 'Now let's change the subject.'

'Do you think Jack and I are meant to be together? How will I know if he's the right one?'

My heart sinks. I have to be careful.

'Maybe relationships need a bit of lots of things: love, friendship, excitement, chemistry, conflict.' I'm pulling words out of a hat. 'I'm not much good at this, as you know. What do you think?'

'I don't know.' She stares despondently into space. 'Sometimes we're such good friends, at others we're worlds apart and I'm unhappy with him. He accepts me for who I am. I like that. Is it enough?'

'I don't know, probably not. When one of us sorts men out we should let the other know. I wish I wasn't so hopeless, for your sake and mine. I wonder how I'll go with Cornelius? I'm trying to be careful. Do you like him?'

'Yes, I think I do. He's friendly and quite attractive. I think he likes you.'

I glance at my watch. 'I'm meant to be over there now having coffee.'

'That's okay. You go. I'll read for a bit and sunbathe.'

I clamber over the lifelines into his cockpit. Cornelius pokes his head out the companionway.

'Sorry I'm late.'

'It's okay. I've had my coffee, yours is in the galley, it'll be cold now.'

We sit together in the empty space of his saloon. 'I really like you,' he begins. 'I'm looking for a long-term relationship. I don't want to waste time – I'm getting old. What are you looking for?'

He's scrutinising me intently. We've hardly known each other five seconds.

'Why, I'm the same. Tell me – what is a good relationship like?' Maybe he can help me and Emily.

'I sailed around the world for ten years with a younger woman, Ursula. We had a good relationship. We loved each other. I know what I want. I've had several good relationships.'

I want to believe him. I need to be with someone who knows about good relationships. I don't. I've never even seen one. I could learn from him.

'I've already fantasised the rest of our lives together,' he tells me. 'You're everything I want in a woman.' His eyes move from dancing to serious, from fun to an intent stare.

I'm flattered. However, I don't want fantasy. I can't afford the luxury of fantasy. I can feel the excitement in me, breaking me up, making it hard to see. I *will* see clearly.

'There's something I need to tell you.' I hold my shaking self, and look at him. 'This is important.' I need to keep it important, to not toss it away for romance.

Cornelius pulls back, as if I'm about to destroy his fantasy. 'I have a spiritual path. It's important to me and will always come first if I have to make a choice. God comes first.'

Cornelius frowns and his eyes go dark. 'I didn't think you believed in God. I thought you were Buddhist.'

'I am, I suppose. I don't like labels.' His eyebrows twitch. 'Buddhism doesn't emphasise personal relationships. Maybe this is one of its limitations.'

He looks uncomfortable and then curious.

'I am interested in the spiritual, you know.'

'I don't expect there will be a problem. Sometimes I need to go away on my own, that's all.

'I had a girlfriend once who went away on retreats. I understand.'

'Dad needs help with things. I must go.'

My position and independence clarified, I stand up, but linger in the galley as my thoughts scramble and run. Cornelius follows close behind me, and as I turn he gently cups my face in his hands. I look shyly into this stranger's eyes. Our lips become sensitive amoebas tasting 'other', but I then pull away and disappear without looking back.

E mily is eagerly awaiting my return and report. 'Well, we kissed,' I grimace. 'I didn't like it – it was too soon.'

She flings her arms up. 'I'm the same. I can't stand men wanting to be close too soon.' Her face looks like she sucked on a lemon. 'I don't even like hugging if it's not right.'

'So I'm not being neurotic? Not about this at least.' I catch her eyes in a broad beam of fun. 'What will I do when you're gone?' I'm so unsure of myself.'

I make plans to keep safe. Cornelius and I will become friends first. I won't throw myself at him like I'm desperate for love, like any angry man will do, like I don't care. I can separate out the 'man' muddle inside me into 'friend' and 'lover'. I'm fooling myself. I know I can't, just like I can't unknot my hair with a toothbrush.

17

Sunlight flickers over Cornelius's bald head and highlights an isolated graft of coarse, crinkly pubic hair, near the front. His bold blue hibiscus flowered shirt hangs loosely over grey boardshorts. Large irregular feet a long way down pause in his well planted sandals.

'Would you like to go out to dinner tonight?' He reaches belatedly for his cap and lights the gas under the coffee. 'There's a good Chinese restaurant in Lautoka.'

'I'd love to.' I'm polite and enthusiastic and swing around to fill myself with the space – tasting, smelling, imbibing the boat, skin prickling with who he is.

Cornelius chats with the taxi driver as if he knows him well, as if they're best friends. I'm not sure whether my question mark will turn into a cross or a tick. Fantasy creeps happy drugs into my brain without me knowing.

In front of a glass of wine and a candle-lit dinner, the bold, flirtatious animal in me takes me over. 'It's too early for us to be kissing. I felt quite uncomfortable afterwards. We'll have to take all of this more slowly.'

I wait for the reaction, the dance. This is fun.

'It was too early for me too. The kiss really shook me up and I had to sit down afterwards to recover.' He pauses. I'm impressed. 'I know what – you can be in charge of this relationship, the pace is up to you.'

'Really?' What a clever reply. 'Okay.'

I'm not sure what it means. It means we have a relationship, that we're on our way. Great. I can relax. We skip the next few pages to the next chapter: how a future together would sketch out. We talk about sailing around the world together, the strongest aphrodisiac

I know, and resting up at Orere Point, a quiet romantic interlude, then we fall headlong into a discussion about failed relationships. We haven't ended up single at forty-seven and sixty-one for no good reason.

The food is lightly-cooked and tasty. 'Mmm, this is so good,' I remark. He doesn't drink much.

I begin on my second glass, not so confident now about who is who and what is what, and my words fly carelessly about. His eyes and smile are inscrutable. He's intense, charming and forthright. That all seems good. Lots of the unknown behind the eyes and words. That's exciting. We talk frankly: probing, enquiring, disclosing. It's a wonderful moment right now, looking across at a new man, soon to be my lover. A whole new body to explore, mind to engage, playmate to go on adventures with. A new start. How wonderful. Soon we'll know each other inside out.

The evening rushes on and the wine dribbles down my throat. I say things better left unsaid, on reflection. He doesn't like them. 'I'm only human', I want to cry, an unstable pack of cards. When I'm shuffled up with another pack I can't tell whether we'll get heart against heart, heart against spade, or spade against spade. I want to be honest but I don't trust myself. I forget the maxim, 'buyer beware', words that would reassure me that, if I'm a vamp and somebody falls for me, I'm not responsible.

I gulp at the wine. We're the only people left. The waiter hovers in the background.

I know I'm too needy. Inside is an unquenchable emptiness. I pretend the opposite. Full of contradiction, that's me. I seem to be available, but I'm not. I drive men crazy. To make it worse, I compete. I was brought up that way. Dad wanted his daughters to be like men. We had to do better than them, beat them at their own game. They were the enemy. Relationships for me are a soup of hard peas.

'Tell me about your life in Hollywood?' I ask, to dress him in its glamour and superficiality and be fascinated by a world I've spent a lifetime ridiculing.

'I went to Beverly Hills High School. My mother wanted me to be in the movies. She was secretary for a big-shot producer. Children of big movie stars were my friends.' He names some but I don't know them.

'I left school to study film production.' He tells his story, clearly, cleanly, full of disappointment and anger. 'I was hijacked by my mother into a career I never wanted.'

I ask for another glass of wine. 'I couldn't succeed, because I didn't understand what I was meant to do and I couldn't stand the back-stabbing. You don't make friends in Hollywood, you make enemies.'

His story is interesting, black almost all the way through. I see a survivor.

'I ended up in ten years of psychoanalysis. My shrink was the one person who loved me. He helped me remake myself into someone other people would like. I learned so much destructive behaviour from my mother – she was a sociopath.'

My wine-soaked brain struggles to evaluate this clearly. Has he really worked through his issues or just tampered with the display? Should I be worried?

I trot to the ladies room and lamely wonder if this is what I want. In my mystical world of light and love I have my 'beloved'. How could human lust match the ecstasy of his embrace and the fine shawl of bliss he wraps around my shoulders? How could the soft breath of a manly chest compare with the deep swell of life itself? I roam within a celestial palace of shimmering moonstone; what need have I to cling to an earthly promise of comfort and adventure. Human warmth is irresistible.

'Do you want coffee or dessert?' He senses I'm drifting away.

'I'm fine. No thanks. Why don't we go for a walk, it's still early.'

'Sure.'

In charge as agreed, I lead him past simple Fijian homes to a trail which follows the rocky shoreline of the harbour. We step carefully in the dark. I wonder if I am lost. 'It's okay, I can smell the piglets, in wire cages. We're on the right track.'

'Really?'

We come out near the abandoned marina. I hold his arm to reassure him. I don't know what he's thinking, but I need to show him who I am. Maybe he's thinking this is slightly unusual. We walk out onto the sine-wave jetty, right down to the far end, and lie on the wooden cladding under the stars. Lautoka 'snow' (sooty smoke from the burning sugar cane refuse) falls softly.

'Isn't this romantic?'

'It's fine,' he murmurs.

In the darkness, our bodies stay apart, building the forcefield, the expectation. Black soot, pigs in cages, a rough trail through the blackness – unconscious symbols poking through. Where are we heading?

'Okay, let's keep going.' I shake away a tipsy tiredness and start up a childish silliness, like I do with Emily, chattering nonsense and throwing my hair around. When I look around the dark street, the warehouses are unfamiliar. Cornelius is following.

'I'm lost.' I tug his arm. 'Let's try this way.' My voice rises to light and nervous and I don't get much of a response, so I skip off in front and kick a beer can towards him. He kicks it back. I can't tell whether he is amused or irritated, I don't know what he wants.

Vuda Point is pronounced Vunda Point. I say the name over and over to myself. A shimmering fishbowl of translucent water – beautiful on the surface, sewage floating just beneath. A surfing friend of Cornelius's fell in by mistake and ended up with festering wounds on his arm. Cold-pressed, organic essential tea-tree oil from my medicine bag didn't help one bit.

I hang onto Emily, to stay steady, and follow her to the resort for our daily swim in chlorinated water followed by a sunbathe on the sun loafers in the bright sunshine and manicured gardens.

'Can you swim the whole length underwater?' she challenges.

We break the water together and speed like torpedoing dolphins to the far end, resurfacing, gasping and spluttering and agreeing that she won. The forward and backward rolls are fun until I forget to hold my nose and become a pygmy whale, snorting phlegmy froth.

From her shoulders I dive down through liquid glass, time slowing under water, ripples of folded light on the painted bottom, anaemic limbs. I tread water as an inner process unfolds flowing skirts and lacy shawls, the instinctive patterning of woman. It all breaks apart into a foolish teenager.

Two weeks zoom past in two days. I move closer on the cushion, until we're touching, our thighs compressed. Then I pause, to normalise this intrusion of male energy, and then breathe deeply, hesitate for the risk, before sinking onto his chest. I look up at him and then turn away to my mind, to create the images and feelings I need to enjoy doing this, flustered, tense and pleased. When his arms fold around me they are warm and alive and when his hands stroke my hair, I become his child come home. I feel my hunger for this warmth, for being held like this, a place to rest in the world, satisfaction in his arms, quietening me, softening me, at peace.

I can't possibly stay here undone by a stranger, and make vapid excuses to stumble up the companionway and escape. I am undone. I go to sleep breathing his smell, his manliness, his voice reverberating through my body, and wake with his arms wrapped around me, my skin alive under his touch. When I climb out onto the deck in the morning light, hugging coffee, I am far away in my drifting body. Women pass with bundles of washing, seabirds cry in the distance, a yacht motors slowly onto its mooring.

Emily flies home tomorrow and we plan a special day together. The dreaming night fades through morning shadow into the bright day.

'Wouldn't it be fun to serenade Cornelius tonight, to say goodbye?' I say.

Emily's voice is lovely and excitement makes me bold. I'm not a singer.

'Well, if you really want to. We'll need to practice. We could wear the new dresses I'm having made. I pick them up this afternoon.'

From scruffy copies of songs from the sixties – songs I sang into the night on the passage over from New Zealand – we choose: 'Scarborough Fair', 'Sailing', 'Streets of London.'

Emily improvises a lively harmony. I hold fast to the simple tune, keeping time with my big toe. Our voices don't blend and lift off into space the way they sometimes do – there's a ragged edge. No time to polish the detail, as we're making a special lunch to surprise Dad when he returns with his bucket of hand-wrung, still soapy washing. He dumps the load in the cockpit to join us at the laden table.

'Well, Emily, I guess you'll be pleased to see Jack? What will you do when you get back?

'I'm not sure.' She lowers her eyes. I pour Dad a glass of wine. 'Maybe we'll go back to Tauranga. Jack's looking for work in the South Island.' She tries to sound more confident than she feels. 'I'm not sure I'll go with him.'

'Relationships aren't always easy.'

She looks at her watch. 'Mum, we have to catch the bus, remember we're going to the movies today.'

At the theatre she stays in charge. 'I'll get the sweets, you get the tickets.'

Monsoon Wedding is a delightfully childlike Indian musical, three happy hours long. Romantic love confronts a traditional Indian family and everyone lives happily ever after. We accept the naivety, the comic-like characters, the ridiculous possibility, the sentimental music. We almost believe in the fairy tale ending – we want to.

'Well, I guess the territory's marked out for me now,' I laugh.

'I'm glad I'm going home. I'm really jealous of Cornelius. You spend so much time with him and I don't know what to do on my own.'

My heart jumps. We'd come back together, in our silliness and adventures and talking. Now I have a new playmate.

'I'm sorry. I thought you were okay.'

We arrive home in the dark, twins in our identical hibiscus-patterned shifts, and creep over to his boat. Torchlight wobbles over the pages above his aft hatch. Our raw voices stay thin and stiff as we scratch at the notes, occasionally stumbling upon the rhythm. Cornelius appears, maybe to stop the noise, and invites us down. He later confessed the music was terrible. He needn't have confessed – I hadn't asked.

Emily leaves early the next morning by taxi, on her own. We hug, she cries, we hug again.

'I like Cornelius,' she tells me.

Then she is gone, back into her own life, far away from me.

I take my coffee up on deck. I wonder what she'll do with the 'me' in her. I sip the last cold dregs. I wish so badly I could reassure her about anything, but I can't. I munch a couple of sweet bananas and swallow tears of sadness and regret, full of my love for her. I pray she goes well and blessings fall on her like rain.

PART FOUR

18

Dad calls down to my bunk where I'm folding jumbled clothes, 'Make sure everything's safely stowed. I want to leave for Musket Cove straight away, before the sun gets high.'

Crumbs smear into grey streaks under my damp cloth. Last bits and pieces squeeze into tight corners.

'Okay, stand by to pull in the lines while Cornelius lets them go. Don't let them float near the propeller.'

Dad hasn't had any luck with his advertisement for a lady companion. Actually he's got cold feet. He's scared of being trundled down a wedding aisle by a Fijian matron.

From a dinghy, the marina helper unties the floating lines, attached to a buoy, that held us off the concrete wall. I coil them neatly.

'See you tomorrow,' Cornelius waves.

Dad reverses smoothly, then eases the throttle forward and turns towards the exit channel. I unhitch and stow fenders that kept us from bumping into *Fantasie*. Soon we're well clear of the rocky coast.

'We can sail to Musket Cove in six hours in this good breeze.' The wind sweeps stale shadows from his face and he stands tall at the helm. 'You can raise the main, all the way.'

I climb up on deck, free again, eyes set on a new horizon. The great rolling beast of the sea rushes past. Cornelius's image casts a film over the sparkling waves. I long to curl myself back up in his arms.

'Dad, the man in my meditation wore a red shirt. Cornelius doesn't have a red shirt. His boat is red, though.' I'm quite sure now our meeting was predestined.

'Well, you certainly came away with romance on your mind. I believe you get what you want. Now, don't sail too close to that marker.' A wobbly stick signals from across the channel. 'The wind's blowing us towards the rocks under the marker, so we need to keep close in this side.' Rocks loom up on this side as well. His brow furrows. 'Actually, the tide may be pulling us towards the rocks this side. I'm not sure what's best. Stay in the middle.'

Dad knows the secret, the Buddha's secret, to steer the middle course.

The browny-blue shallow water is clear in the midday sun, so I can steer safely through the middle.

Inside I'm all caught up on a hook of longing. I want to be back in his arms, resting on his chest, his child come home. The hunger in me won't let go now I've let it out.

Dad noses into a tight cleft between two coral fingers, close in to shore.

'Okay, drop the anchor – about forty feet should do.'

We're back at Musket Cove with a new set of dinghies jostling and jumping on the rising tide.

'I'll buy sausages and meet you at the bar. I'm going for a short walk,' I call as I turn away.

I walk as I always do – to hold myself together, aloof and alone, safe in myself, – deep breath, short breath, heart pounding, diffusing what was disturbing, finally safe.

Back at the three-dollar bar, exclusively rewrapped in my aloneness, I drop foiled potatoes into a nest of red-hot embers. Dad throws back rum, I sip wine and roll the sausages and push hard potatoes further into the embers. I gulp for breath – a fish out of water. I won't start conversations I'm already bored with. Raining chatter dribbles into puddles at my feet. This spit of reclaimed land is far too human for me. Suddenly I remember and help arrives: I should be watching my moods and memories, I'm not meant to be sunk by them. Everything changes in that instant of recollection, my mind lets go and spreads out wide, free from any point of view. Life gets to dance while I trickle runny butter into our mushy potatoes and join the circus.

Back on *Dream-maker*, still enjoying this spacious mind, Dad and I relax in the saloon with cups of tea and legs spread out. Water sloshes and slaps the hull; a cool breeze wafts in through the darkness; dinghies approach and retreat like noisy mosquitoes. I consciously start to let my mind alone, like before, intrigued by where it might go now I'm very quiet, what it might encounter, what it might tell me about life as it spreads way out. It's like I'm untying myself, the end of a balloon, to let my mind free, compressed air expanding into the space all around.

I settle back, scrunched pillow in my lower back, cushion supporting my upper back, observing in this new way. This new perspective is without a boundary – it has lost the compelling reference of me. I start seeing directly into the dream of Dad and me sailing backwards and forwards across the ocean. The minute detail comes into focus. Everything we do, every movement we make, is an exquisite, perfect expression of the whole, the finest music. Dad strokes his mosquito bite as an integrated response to everything around him, both spontaneous and preordained, perfect. We never stray from the part we are playing in this dance of life. Dad turns the page of his book and looks over to me, following an imperative, polished to perfection in the finest detail. As he raises his hand and turns his head to adjust the reading light, everything inside the boat moves and turns with him, making way, tuning him – a melody of a thousand different parts. How could it not be like this? He can't move unless the air gives way to make his movement possible, unless the cushion remoulds itself. They are in agreement. I can't lift my journal unless my journal allows me to lift it. This might sound ludicrous but it's perfectly obvious in this moment. The whole of life is willing everything we do, participating and supporting us. A global mind is willing this dance. The individual mind is the illusion.

He arrives! Grouped up with his surfing friends under the painted light bulbs, I glow and bubble under his hand reassuringly on my back, in the limelight as his new girlfriend.

Before the lights go dim, a shadow of strain buckles my face, the refrain, the taut rope. 'Can we go for a walk?'

'Sure,' he replies, his voice edged with surprise.

Hand in hand, through the dark night, we trace sandy pathways past suburban resorts, pathways well worn by me now. Restaurants are emptying at the far end of the island. I walk like walking will absolve me, hold me together, banish my demons. The dinghy dock is almost empty of humanity when we return to our dinghy and motor back to *Dream-maker*. Cornelius kisses me a tender goodnight before buzzing directly back to *Fantasie*.

This afternoon Cornelius and Dad talked about us sailing around Cape Horn and up to the Mediterranean. This is one of the greatest sailing challenges there is! Cornelius wants to do it with me! I listened, nodding like a wobbly-headed doll, my insides in total disarray and excitement.

I'm walking through suburban streets cluttered with houses – weatherboard and brick, single-storey matchbox houses on flat dry lawn. The odd standard rose or ornamental tree, wilting marigolds and petunias just survive in the dry soil. A light is on inside a house, a long way away from me. The street is always shadowy, even in the afternoon. I don't exist anywhere, bleached like the concrete underfoot, the ragged uncut edges of grass, the clogged mud stuck in the grates of the street drains.

Cornelius calls 'Good morning' as his dinghy bumps gently up against *Dream-maker*.

'Come aboard,' I shout, scampering up to take his painter. 'Dad and I are just having coffee. Would you like some?' I flutter like a butterfly, alighting briefly, shivering inside.

'Sure.' He clambers aboard and fixes on Dad. 'Roger, how are you? I like your spot. Not many captains would be game to anchor this close to the coral.'

Dad moves involuntarily, to dissipate the pleasure he feels. 'Ah, well, I've anchored here many times over the years. So you're off scuba diving. You have excellent weather.'

'That's right – no wind, clear sky.'

I smile at Cornelius. 'I'll go put on my togs and get my snorkelling gear.'

Dad becomes serious. 'Alice has never been scuba diving. She doesn't know anything about the danger or the equipment or the theory.'

Cornelius stays cool. 'Roger, I appreciate your concern. I've taught at least twenty people to dive over the years. We'll go ashore first so she can get the hang of the gear. We're not going very far or deep. She'll be fine with me.'

I listen while the kettle boils. Dad hassled me last night about the danger.

Cornelius's dinghy is full of bottles, vests, stuff I have no idea about but want to learn.

'Don't worry, we'll be fine.' I toss a parting wave to Dad. Of course I will be – I love this sort of thing.

Cornelius's thighs limp out of his bleached maroon togs, hollow where the muscle is wasting away. This will be me in a few years. A ragged black T-shirt hangs over his bulging gut. Today he's my hero because he's taking me on an adventure.

'We'll go in here, this side of the point, where it's sandy and shallow.' He unwinds the throttle to slow us down. Wake rides up from behind and shovels us on shore. Yeh! I'm on an adventure I haven't had to make happen myself! Maybe all those years of being the man in my life are over. The sand is dazzling bright in the sunlight and slippery underfoot when we step out to paddle the dinghy in through water gently slapping the wobbly sides.

Cornelius gives me his full attention. 'I've clipped everything together this time; you can see how it goes later. Here's your vest.'

I poke at the shapeless mass.

'The tanks strap in like this. They're heavy.' He clips and pulls some straps around my waist to secure the vest and tank. I wobble like a lifeless doll being dressed.

'This is the respirator.' Nothing makes much sense yet. 'This is how you breathe.'

I try it. 'Now put on your weights, they'll balance the buoyancy in the vest.'

I concentrate. I don't want to make a mistake or forget anything. I focus really hard.

'This is the breather for releasing air from your vest. This is where you blow to increase your buoyancy. Breathe in to fill your vest with air and let the air out like this, so you can sink in the water.' It seems complicated. He repeats the instruction. 'This dial tells you how much air you have left. One tank will last about half an hour.'

I swim around in the shallows, practising until I am no longer confused. I pretend it's easy – to myself and to him.

'You're a natural,' he compliments me when I surface. 'You're ready for the real thing. Let's go out to the reef.'

I wriggle and shrug my arms out of the vest, glowing with pride, then lift the air tanks and weight belt into the dinghy, showing no sign of effort, even though they're heavy. We motor away, me at the helm, face into spray bursting onto my skin. I don't want him to see me because I can't stop smiling.

We bob, anchored through 20 feet of crystal-blue glass into sand. Smoky sapphire blue covers the heavens. Cornelius lifts my air tank, I put the respirator in my mouth, tighten all the straps and fall backwards off the boat. A wall of intense claustrophobia rushes at me. I need to take all the stuff off right now and get out to where I can breathe real air. I can't. I breathe through my panic, push it away and head down. Impossibly sharp pain shoots through my ears. I swallow hard, then block my nose and breathe hard, to balance the pressure on both sides of my ear drums. The pain gets worse. I blow air into my vest and float up until the pain lessens, then dive again. I float up and dive down, over and over, until the pressure inside my ears equalises and I can get all the way to the bottom.

Lobsters twitch their feelers and poke nervously from deep crevices. A turtle glides past like a slow-moving frisbee. Great coral umbrellas stretch towards golden blue light filtering down. Cornelius comes up behind me and takes my hand. We paddle along together. He gathers starfish and sea cucumbers for me to touch and turn over. I get brave enough to stroke the feathery seaweeds and soft corals. Colourful fish dart in and out of the coral, nibbling the edges. They're weightless, like us. Water has made us all slow and graceful. Our movements seem so peaceful, natural, effortless. I was this watery movement the first nine months of my life. Experience of harsh dry air came later.

Cornelius had instructed me that scuba divers don't use their arms to swim, so I don't – I only paddle my feet. I paddle into a growing experience of exquisite order and sweep into philosophical sea eggs. It's all so harmonious. Everything fits in. Nothing is trying to be different, stand out, go it alone. There's no 'trying hard' here, no shoulds or oughts, rights or wrongs.

I follow Cornelius's flippers and his spent bubbles trickling to the surface. We break back through into planetary air together.

'Why did you swim away on your own?' Cornelius asks. 'It's important to stay together. You're a natural, though,' he grins.

'I'm sorry. We do everything together now,' I lie.

Our dinghy zooms us back to *Dream-maker* to reassure Dad, and then to *Fantasie* for our first night together. I'll be brushing my teeth on his boat for the first time.

Encouraged by incense and soft music, Cornelius turns out the light and strokes me gently. My hand reaches down. His penis is soft, too soft. He does come though, in my mouth. I lie awake while he drifts off to sleep. First dawn trickles through the hatch and he rolls over for loving. He kisses me until I drown in shivering bursts of bliss.

'Do you feel this too?' I whisper. 'I feel like we've known each other forever. I've come home to you.'

He kisses me until I'm a squirming babe in his arms and he is my boundless, loving mother. I become all given to him, drifting with no idea who I am or where I'm bound.

Yesterday, I challenged him to a wrestling match to test his strength against mine. We pushed and pulled, tumbling on the hard lawn, the way I did with my Dad and all my boyfriends when I was young. From today on, in the warm sun, anchored in a blue sea with a tickle of a breeze, I will stop my persistent searching through, clambering over, tunnelling under. I will give up to the gentle currents floating Cornelius and me together. Wind whispers in the rigging. The boat rocks gently inside our bodies, sinking us in its translucent waves of soft light. I don't ever want to leave this space. It's like we are swimming together, back through time into that place where sea birds and flittering fish first started out. I slip away into a peaceful, mysterious ocean. We become like water babies wriggling through each other to a place underneath all the disappointments and hurts that hardened us in the noonday sun. We are as soft and sweet as a new dawn.

'Hi, Dad – just coming to see how you are.'

He's folded up in the saloon, listening to some music.

'Shall I make us a cup of tea?'

His boat's a mess and he's been drinking. An empty whiskey bottle pokes from an overflowing rubbish bag and another half-empty one sits on the floor.

'Why don't I make us some lunch?' I go into the galley and put water on to boil.

'I'm pretty bored, I have to admit.' He tries not to be reproachful. 'When I get back to Lautoka, I'm going to advertise again and find a sailing companion.'

'That's a great idea. Do you want some help with writing the ad?' I hunt around for a tin of tuna.

'Yes, I do. I've almost finished the draft. You know better than me what women like to hear.' He lights a cigarette and looks up at a peek of sky bobbling through the companionway. 'I'm not very optimistic, mind you.'

'Here's some pasta and tuna sauce.' I pass a small bowl, embarrassed about our state of affairs.

'I need to be careful. If Angela finds out she'll be wild.' He pauses briefly to tuck in his shirt. 'I don't know what else to do. Angela's a liability on a boat. She was seasick all the way over last time. I'm not up to getting her into and out of a dinghy. Didn't put her off, though.'

'Dad, she loves you. Why don't you ask her to fly over?'

'She wouldn't come, not now.'

A neatly scribbled list of affirmations sits under his pen and a dog-eared copy of *The Seven Habits of Highly Effective People* bides its time on the navigation table.

'I'm going now. I expect you for dinner. We're eating about six.'

Cornelius greets me from the cockpit. 'How's your father?'

The dinghy bumps against the hull. He doesn't seem to notice – that's good. I bump against his barrel chest and hunt for his mouth.

'He's not doing well. I don't know what to do.'

Cornelius moves away to stare across the windy harbour. 'I understand his aloneness, I've been horribly alone on my boat, going ashore and sitting in a bar every night, waiting for someone to talk to. There aren't many single women around marinas. Actually there are a few more now. You have the pick of single-handers here. There's not much competition and they all want a woman.'

I smile. 'Well, I have you.' I burrow back into his chest. 'Let's go downstairs.'

'Are you serious about sailing around Cape Horn with me?' I ask when I pop up for breath.

'Sure. We get to wear a golden ring in our ear. Which ear depends on which way round the Cape we sail. Let's look at the atlas. Maybe we'll stop at Morocco on the way.'

I squirm with delight. 'My kids will have to fly over to join us. That's okay isn't it?'

'Sure. A ready-made family climbing over my boat and girlfriend!'

We pore over the atlas, tracing ragged coastlines of exotic countries, planning our route. He knows I'm holding on to this sailing adventure the way he holds onto my body.

'I wouldn't do it alone, though. The company of men in marinas gets boring. Men don't get close to each other. We talk about boats and share sailing stories.' He sits up and stares straight into my eyes, his hands on my thighs. 'The only place I can share who I am is with you.' I shiver at the tunnel of light in his eyes. 'With you I can be vulnerable and real. Harsh salt winds, ragged lines, callused hands and rusty bolts make your softness extraordinary. I won't let go easily.' He grimaces at a sudden pain streaking down his leg and hobbles to the medicine cupboard.

'My leg's getting worse. Now my foot's going numb. I'm falling apart. Why now?'

I stare after him, my voice reduced to a squeak. 'Do you think a hottie will help? It must be your back. Are you okay? I could show you some yoga exercises to strengthen and tone your back muscles.'

The interior darkens as the boat swings away from the sun. He limps to the for'ard bunk, defeated.

'I've always wanted to try yoga. Fancy meeting a yoga teacher. Not right now, though.' I can't tell whether he's grimacing from the pain or the thought of yoga.

'I hope this isn't serious,' he continues to moan. 'I've never been unwell. I don't have any medical insurance – I've never needed it.'

19

*F*antasie realigns itself to the changing wind and tide, following all the other boats in here, which is just as well because we're packed in like sardines.

Dad putters over the lumpy water for his morning coffee. 'We can't sail back to Lautoka today – there's too much wind. I'm sorry.'

Cornelius looks at me intently. 'The sea's too rough for us to go scuba diving. The light won't reach the coral.'

'Another day of rest then,' I beam, so they can relax. We sit and chat about small things until sea and sky grow empty spaces between us.

'Well, I'll go potter on some small jobs.' Dad puts down his cup. 'Thanks for the coffee.'

'Dad, I want to go ashore later,' I call after him. 'We'll pick you up.'

I gather up the cups and follow Cornelius inside.

I can't get away and I don't want to. His long fingers trace my body, as myself; his intoxicatingly sweet breath trickles into my lungs, as me; his deep voice cascades through my quivering body, delighting every wobble of my internal landscape. What's to be done with me? The boundaries are no longer clear. When I had babies, I didn't know who was who in our vulnerable intimacy. I was full of feelings I couldn't name. I slept cuddled around their porcelain bodies, sunk in the mystery of identity. I'm the same now. When I lifted a new baby into my arms I couldn't take my eyes away, I couldn't stop looking, smelling, touching – my baby, me, tumbling together.

I leap from his arms to a point of view, separated out, only to enjoy burying back down, losing myself in his flesh, claiming his love with my mouth. Elegant ideas, spooled into complicated sentences

and turns of phrase, fly across the room to impress and challenge, to
delight in the other. I consider his response, who he is, critically and
objectively. He thinks clearly, he has style, he has good manners, he's
interesting, he's intelligent. He gets lots of ticks.

'What about politics?' I ask.

'I'm ashamed of being American.' The few hairs on his head bristle.
'The invasion of Iraq is disgraceful. I don't fly my American flag
now – most Americans don't – it may be dangerous.' Sixty years of
American pride is crumbling, his guts are leaking, his back is giving
way. 'China will be the next superpower – they're who we should be
looking out for.'

I tick the politics box.

'Tell me more about your therapy?'

He puts down his tea and softens against a cushion, for his back.
His voice turns deep and hard. 'It took years of therapy to find out
my mother didn't love me. She didn't have my best interests at heart.'

We agree on the psychological foundation of emotional dysfunction.
I tick that box. Mostly we're on the same page. Can I imagine us
together? We seem to understand each other. I like who I am with
him: he challenges me, he makes me accountable for what I say – I
can't be sloppy. I'm being as objective as I can.

Cornelius leaves the galley where he's taken to nibbling crackers.
His dark shadow swoops down and sweeps me up, crushing me
against him. We tumble down as he rips at my clothes and consumes
me with his lips and hands, dissolving in my fragility. I become
lost in whirling ecstasy, fuelled by whispers and tender caresses. I
tremble at his voice; I quiver under his touch. His fiery passionate
desperation will at last make me his woman. His penis is finally
hard and he slides deep inside me. I fade into a great circle of
white light, lost to the intensity. He gasps his relief. My eyes stare
blankly at the ceiling, unsure of what has happened. I can't name
my broken, ownerless, wobbly, shattered state. Cornelius rests next
to me, peaceful, nested in my arms. I want to stand up and declare
what has happened. Our union feels world-shakingly important.
Maybe it's just sex.

'Let's go outside and have a boat lesson,' I finally suggest when we've equilibrated to moderate. 'I have so much to learn. We could make a start.'

He follows me up, relieved for the vertical perspective and delightfully muddled by our passion and his performance. The day is full-on glare, solid chunky shapes, blinding reflections, boats bucking and prancing at anchor, wind freshening. At the harbour entrance the waves tumble as an outgoing tide runs into an onshore wind. In here we're protected by the reef. My feet hit solid cockpit, solid movement, not formless inner gyrations. Sun burns my shoulders.

'First you need to know about self-tailing winches. Your Dad doesn't have them. With a self-tailing winch you'll be able to furl the headsail on your own.' Cornelius puts the winch handle in place and cranks it a couple of times.

'These running back stays support the main.' His hand hangs on rope running from the mast to the back of the boat. 'Your Dad doesn't have them either. The upwind stay is kept tensioned. The downwind stay stays slack. When we go about or gybe we have to re-tension them.'

'What do 'gybing' and 'going about' mean?' I'm confused. My head shakes involuntarily, wobbling me down to my toes. 'Back stays? I hardly know what ordinary stays are.' I grab the rod rigging for support. I'm being far too honest.

Cornelius's eyes narrow and darken. 'I thought you knew how to sail?'

'Well, I do, sort of. I can sail Dad's boat, but I still have lots to learn.' I grab the lifeline with my other hand, wishing I'd never suggested a lesson. 'I'm good at things once I've learned them.' I frown seriously, pulling in my chin for dignity. 'I learn slowly but I need to practice and try things out in my own way to learn.'

That confession would have set off an Epurb (an emergency location device) in a lesser man, but not Cornelius.

'Okay, come up and check the main. There are two winches. I use the large one, but it's over-powered so you have to be careful not to overstretch the leech.'

I wonder, but I won't ask. Is the leech the boom side or the mast side of the sail, or the hypotenuse in between? Overstretch the leech? It must be the mast side of the sail. Whew!

'Always look up when you're raising the main, to make sure it's not caught on anything.'

I change tack and boom a glorious compliment. 'You'll be an excellent teacher. You're a professional sailor and this is a real racing yacht. The mast is so tall compared to *Dream-maker*'s.'

Cornelius grimaces. 'Come, I'll show you the stays and turnbuckles. I have different kinds, so you can learn from the differences.'

I trot after him. I like this masculine world, separated out and practical. Turnbuckles connect the stays to the chainplates. Chainplates bolt to the hull. The relationships are clear and straightforward. Together they hold up the mast.

I can't wait to go sailing together. Rod rigging is superior to wire rigging; it doesn't stretch. Cornelius scratches his head; he can't make me out at all.

M y grey bubble of a dinghy bounces me back and forth between *Dream-maker* and *Fantasie* and then ashore, when I need to go alone. I row to keep solid, to stop disintegrating into soft mush. This mush is disconcerting. Nothing outside is solid or very real anymore. This is what so much love making has done to me. I wonder if this is what I was like in the womb. Diffuse light and undulating softness. Maybe this was my earliest experience, before the harsh air jolted my ordinary senses into action.

'Cornelius, I'm going ashore for a walk. I'll meet you by the store in a couple of hours.'

'Sure. It's quite choppy out there. That dinghy of yours is pretty lightweight.' Straightforward and clear, he knows who he is. I wish I did. 'I'll take you in if you like?'

'I'll be fine.' I push off *Fantasie*'s belly with my oar, before he changes his mind – feet on the painter which traces rough squiggles in the belly of the dinghy, pressing into the soft plastic base. I pull firmly on the short aluminium oars. The bubble bounces and bobs over the surface, swinging towards shore. A large craft roars up, reduces it throttle and sends a flotilla of waves towards me. The bearded captain calls, 'Would you like a tow?'

'Thanks for offering, but I enjoy rowing. I like the exercise.'

He roars past, bouncing me around all over again in his wake. Spray flying over the bow drenches me so I lick the salt from my face, and brush the dripping hair from my eyelashes. Being alone in the sea like this is the best.

My dinghy continues to bounce about tied up at the dinghy dock. With briskly slapping jandals flicking up sand, I start walking again – a new route behind the resorts, past a rubbish dump and idle machinery, around to a small scrappy jungle breathing out fresh air. My circumnavigation returns me to bulldozers dredging soil for a new waterway, turning nature into money. Pretty shells poke from the mud. I take stock of where I am – I'm a jumbled-up mess that I don't understand and I'm out of control.

As we clamber on board *Dream-maker* Dad boasts, 'I'm cooking cordon bleu tonight.'

His words run together, his face is rosy. He's pushed books and papers to the side of the table, to make room for the food. Chicken sizzles on the stove, ingredients for a large salad are wilting on the table and scrubbed potatoes soak in dirty sink water.

'I'll pour you a rum and coke.'

He picks up a half empty bottle and turns to Cornelius.

'Well, Cornelius, how've you been today? How's your leg?' He tops up our glasses with coke. 'I've been listening to the BBC. I'm glad we can get it here. They're saying that the invasion of Iraq is all about oil. It's not to do with terrorism and Sadam at all. Bush is lying to the world.'

Cornelius sits down to stretch out his bad leg. 'Yes, Roger, I couldn't agree more. I know you don't like Americans. Now you've good reason not to.' He walks a fine line. He likes Roger and he must be seen to like him. Dad and I follow him to the table. I worry about the potatoes.

'Dad, why is it you don't like Americans?'

'Hump,' Dad mutters. He doesn't want to admit his prejudice. 'Well, in business I've been cheated by Americans and, during the war when they were stationed in New Zealand, they seduced all the girls. Kiwi blokes didn't get a look in. The American soldiers were confident, charming and wealthy. Cornelius, you seem okay, though. It's not personal.'

'Thanks, Roger.'

'Dad, I'll put the potatoes on if you like and check the chicken.'

'No, no, you're my guests tonight.' He returns to the galley.

I tidy up the salad. Cornelius is charming. Dad becomes more garrulous as the evening flows. Cornelius is patient and attentive. I become jealous of Dad getting all the attention. I don't like the feeling, because Dad needs this attention. Hours roll by – I'm totally bored. 'Men's talk' is tediously superficial. I clean up. Steam from the boiling kettle hisses through the galley. I pass around instant coffee in tea-stained mugs and slump down to wait it out.

We finally say goodbye and cross the moonless night back to *Fantasie*. I put the kettle on again. My dependence on tea amuses Cornelius. I tell him about the confusion, my hurts and betrayals with men, excited by the risk I'm taking. Cornelius has lived through so much loneliness, I'm sure he won't be careless or offhand with me. I jump around the saloon, blurting out everything. I can't help it – I don't want secrets between us. I'm looking for unconditional acceptance. I want to confess and be absolved. I rush into his arms when I need reassurance and push away when I'm ready to go on. He listens carefully. I sound dangerous. I sound too much like his mother. And isn't that the hook.

He smiles ruefully. 'You say that Max was never there for you, but it sounds like you're the one who kept running away.'

I start at his sudden resistance, knocked off my perch by this other point of view. I've frightened him off. I have no perspective on my situation. I explode into bubbles of sweat.

'Am I too dangerous to be trusted?'

He holds me close, like he knows what I am going through, and whispers, 'You can always depend on me. You'll be the one to determine the outcome of this relationship.'

He strokes my hair.

'How can you be so sure?'

The fantasy of 'always' slips by. My right eye sees reality and my left eye sees fantasy and the views don't match. I don't see out of my right eye much, so I don't know. The fuzz of the two views intersecting is my fear. The fuzz is the fuses blowing, because the fantasy my child-mind is growing doesn't have real people in it with different points of view and agendas of their own.

He kisses me ever so gently and snuggles his way down into my flesh. We try to make love but he is too soft. I feel his anxiety and frustration.

'It's okay, penises and hearts have a way of their own.' I hug him confidently in the dark. The boat rocks us gently back and forth, away from our troubles. 'Our hearts are singing to each other,' I reassure him. 'They're simply children peeping out under grown-up skirts, sharing smiles and laughter. Our hearts don't care about these other things.'

He kisses me again and carries me away with his unimaginable gentleness. My head rocks in his hand. She's crazy, but it doesn't matter, her body is all that matters, he's thinking.

The middle of the night turns dark and tortured.

'The pain in my leg is unbearable,' he yells, reaching for the light switch. 'A sharp stabbing pain is shooting all the way down.'

I fill him another hot water bottle.

'I still can't sleep,' he moans a bit later on. 'I don't want to keep you awake – I'm going to the saloon.'

He leaves without a kiss. I sink heavily into the turmoil of my disclosures. He tosses and turns far away from me. I pull up the covers so they keep out the cold. They don't – I'm cold all through. I've been abandoned. He can't stand the pain, what pain? I'm someone he knows. I don't want him to wake up in the morning, protected from her in an offhand way. I want him for me; I want him to delight in me. I've slipped into being like a child. I don't know how to be a woman. I can be his child; I can stay a child. I can't – I need to grow up. I don't know how. I won't grow back into the woman I was.

'Let's do some yoga. Some simple exercises might help your back.' I suggest, after our morning coffee in the cockpit.

We take opposite sides of the saloon, perched on the dark green squabs.

'We'll do the cat/cow first. Onto your hands and knees.' He scrunches up his face like a child starting school. 'Watch me first. Do the movement with the breath – breathe in as you arch your back and then breathe out as you bow it. Keep your awareness in your spine. If you do the exercise in a distracted way it won't help. It's the awareness that counts.'

His body moves in a saggy and flabby way. I won't say anything.

'Now lie down on your tummy, hands at your shoulders and slowly lift your head. Arch your back and breathe into your chest. Don't let your pelvis lift up. Hold for three breaths, then lower, unrolling your spine slowly.' He looks pretty stiff. He's hardly moving. 'We'll do that three times.'

'Now roll onto your back and bring your knees up to your chest. That's right. Roll gently and wriggle your spine from side to side. That's good.' He looks like a dead pillow. 'How was that?'

'The exercises were too hard. I'm not an advanced student – I need something much more gentle.' He looks disgusted.

'Really. They were pretty simple.'

'No, I've seen simpler exercises.'

Cornelius comes ashore so he can shower his yoga sweat away and check his emails. I wait under a coconut palm, watching Fijians at volleyball. They leap after the ball, knocking against each other, laughing uproariously. Sands sprays from brown flesh boldly bared to the sun. The ball flies down the beach to where tourists lie like upturned turtles under striped umbrellas. Bronzed yachties, piled up with groceries, trickle from the general store.

This world can't be real. I never would have dreamed this. My life for so long was driving along a clogged motorway to work, tired before every day started. How did I get to be on an endless romantic holiday? I know the bubble will pop and dump me back on the motorway. I'm floating in a bubble, bobbing over a dark unfriendly ocean. It's going to pop, pop, pop. These shimmering reflections are telling me who I am, I am, I am. Let me out. I'm trapped inside. This is fantasy. People poke my bubble from the outside, trying to get in. There's no one inside but me.

'Dad, we're ready.' I call. 'I've got chicken, rice and a salad.'

He appears from the companionway. 'How are you, Cornelius?'

I look carefully to see how he is as he climbs down into the waiting dinghy.

At the three-dollar bar I rummage about in my bag and look up with a "how stupid can you get" look.

'I've left the food behind. I'll go and pick it up.'

Cornelius starts at my suggestion. 'You don't know how to drive my dinghy. Are you sure?' He looks at me intently, then turns to Dad. 'Roger, what do you think?'

Dad tosses his reply: 'She'll be fine.'

I need some time alone and I like a challenge. Cornelius's outboard is ten horsepower; Dad's is two and a half.

'I'll be fine.' I set off cockily down to the pontoon before Cornelius can change his mind.

I untie the dinghy, gingerly start the motor and steer slowly out through the narrow channel, not too close to either side. I give the engine a little more power and immediately zigzag out of control, then breathe forcefully and slow down. I can't see Dad's boat in the dark and creep along, checking out the hulls until *Dream-maker* looms into view. How do I come alongside? I bounce into the hull and the motor stops by itself. Good. My heart pounds as I tie up and clamber aboard to get the potatoes and Dad's jacket.

My legs turn to jelly. I put the engine in neutral and pull the start cord. The dinghy shoots away. Obviously I missed neutral. I zigzag over to *Fantasie*, revving and slowing, pushed all over the place by my wake. I turn a couple of circles, shaking inside, before settling on a plan for the best approach. I bounce against the hull, side on this time, while the motor screams and tries to drag me off. When I press the red button, the motor stops. I breathe deeply until my heart slows down. I'm way out of my depth; I'd much rather be rowing. I pick up the chicken – now I have all our food. I did it!

I set off again, zooming steadily to shore, confident enough to fade into my dream of romance. I steer blindly across to the other side of the narrow entrance. The dinghy suddenly stops moving. What! Totally disorientated, I take ages to sort out what's happening. The engine roars, screams, shrieks. I'm aground. In a total panic, I rev the motor some more to get me off. The engine roars and roars, faster and faster driving the propeller into the sand. What can I do? In a flash of inspiration I stop the motor. I'm petrified. What if I've broken something expensive? I sit in the dark until I stop shaking. Nobody's going to rescue me. Eventually I think to climb into the cold tide and push off the sandy shelf. Still shaking, I clamber back in and pull the starter cord, not knowing what to expect. The engine starts. I can't tell if it sounds any different. I creep slowly back to the dinghy dock, tie up and return to Dad and Cornelius with our food, jelly legs firming up on the hard ground.

Cornelius smiles, relieved to see me. 'How did you go?'

'I was fine,' I lie weakly, with a laugh.

The bar is full of yachties and Dad soon finds company over a rum or two, leaving me and Cornelius to cook. I snuggle safely back into his arms, poking the chicken sizzling over the fire. The soft light, sandy floor, wooden tables and jostling crowd are our prize. His deep voice reverberates through me. We've been together through lifetimes, stretching back as far as the beginning of time. Shape-changing, victorious, we found each other again. We are heroes of the boundless universe.

Time is chasing us. I am sailing back to Lautoka with Dad; Cornelius is sailing to Vuda Point, close by. We will be apart! I await my sentence in the cockpit, hands tightly around a mug of strong black coffee. Cornelius is below cooking. My fingers pick senselessly at a plate of eggy fried bread. The impossibility of this very moment sweeps over me, like a gigantic darkness passing in front of the sun. Paralysed, I watch the universe turn on the point of the cockpit, a great spinning top whirling into space. This moment – eggy bread and morning light –is hugely significant and yet it is utterly meaningless. Bubbled forth from nothing, to nothing it will return. A blink and it's over: light returned to dark. A primal jolt of terror hits me. Like a baby, when I close my eyes the world will be gone. I shake my head several times to get back to normal.

'Here's some more toast.' Cornelius passes the plate and stares into my eyes. 'You look different this morning.' He stares into my face. 'You have the eyes of a wise bovine extraterrestrial.'

'Do I?' I reply with a crackly, dry throat.

20

As *Fantasie* threads through the coral ahead of us, Dad calls, 'Something's wrong with the voltage regulator. Can you take the wheel?' He disappears downstairs. I steer through the coral and rock.

'You need to keep our speed down. Watch the dial doesn't go over 8,000 rpm.' Cornelius slips further in front.

'What's going on?' I ask. 'We normally motor at 15,000 rpm.'

'The voltage regulator isn't reducing the power to the batteries. They might overcharge. There's nothing we can do but motor slowly.'

I turn the wheel to counteract the wind, as *Fantasie* slips over the horizon. Dad's voice breaks into my misty unformed longing. A longing, deeper than Cornelius but drawn out by him, a longing to be united, surrendered, transported beyond myself, a longing for oblivion, wholeness.

'I'll take the wheel while you pull up the main. The puff of wind might help.'

I jump with a start. Human touch is irresistibly sweet. Like sugar, it's addictive, highly prized in evolutionary terms. The touch of my beloved doesn't have this sharp edge of craving.

'Sure.'

I pull up the main with extra care, making sure nothing is caught. I check the tension on the leech, cleat the halyard, coil the line fastidiously. I check that everything on deck is in order.

The wind dies and our motor turns slowly. Late afternoon, sun-dried and hungry, we chug into Lautoka.

'Dad, what do think of Cornelius? He's a pretty interesting person don't you think?'

'Um, yes, I suppose so. I'll see if I can get the news.'

He pours a drink.

'Those photos in his boat, taken from his trip around the world – they're good, aren't they?'

'Um, yes. Ah, here it is.' He turns the radio up loud.

I put sausages on to fry. Maybe Dad is jealous of me. I peel a couple of spuds and toss the skins into the tide. Maybe he doesn't think Cornelius is good enough for me. Something's wrong. Maybe he's just lonely. He's sick of Cornelius. I slice the beans and put them in with the potatoes. Maybe it's everything mixed up – a mix that requires many stiff whiskeys.

'Here Alice, can you have a look at this?'

I sit down and look at his new ad for a sailing companion.

'It's too wordy and too extravagant. Do you think the right kind of person will answer it?'

'It's my only chance.'

'You should take this out and this too. There, that should do.' I read it out loud to test the flow. 'Yes, that's good now – I hope it works.'

'So do I. What else can I do? I'm lonely. Cornelius arranged for me to use the phone of the woman at the email café. Before you arrived he advertised in the local paper and had lots of replies.'

I fall into bed wide awake. Cornelius usually kisses me to sleep. How can I fall asleep on my own without his beautiful hands caressing me? How is he, without my little body snuggled against his? Why has he become so precious to me? Because I've turned him into my beloved, that's why. I've mixed them up. I roll over in bed. The love I feel is real, but we aren't. How strange. I sit up in the dark so I can think more clearly. I have fallen into the love that ripples the world alive and I want to stay there. I smile sheepishly. I don't understand the human part of love; I never did. I don't care for who he is as a man. I probably wouldn't like him. I don't like men.

I get up and make a midnight cup of cocoa, so I can consider this important matter: the mystical embrace, perfection, beyond pain or sorrow. The ordinary world has consequences, responsibilities and duties. I don't know the point of this grownup world, but it's where I belong. I sip my cocoa, with more sugar to give me energy. I'm starting to get overexcited. The mystical mind is narcissistic – that's the problem. It doesn't break the world into other points of view, other people. I need to find out how I got so lost inside myself, why I didn't separate out properly.

I turn out the light and snuggle back down under my blanket. I worry about seeing Cornelius tomorrow. We will be separated. Will he appear ordinary? That disquieting ordinary that hovers and makes an appearance every now and then. Oh dear, I must try and sleep now – it's very late – but how, how to go to sleep without him.

'Here's a cup of tea, Alice. Time to wake up.'

'I don't want to wake up, I'm tired.' I rummage around for my watch and peek, one eye open. 'Is it really eight o'clock?' I drag myself into sitting. 'What time do you want to go to Lautoka?' I slurp warm milky tea onto my T-shirt.

'I'd like to go early, as soon as we've had breakfast.'

'I have to check my emails,' I grump. 'I don't want to. I don't want anything to take me away from here.' Dad looks at me like I'm mad. 'I'm worried about my houses. I promised to keep in touch with my kids, so I will.'

I gulp down the last mouthful. I knew I'd find it hard to stop running and it is.

'Well, I'm looking forward to seeing who's written to me,' he responds. 'You'll love hearing from your children. Don't be so silly.'

I turn my back so I can dress somewhat privately. 'Remember, I'm bussing straight from town to Cornelius's boat at Vuda Point. I expect to see you there in a couple of days.'

My clothes are in lumps all over the place. What should I take? I'm losing the plot. I fill a bag. I'm tired. My body can't take any more love-making – the voltage regulator stopped working ages ago.

We set out in the morning sun. Dad's breath is short and jerky. My thighs slap the loose maroon sarong which is a bad match with my brown leather sandals. We're both hidden under ungainly sunhats. Sometimes I dress smartly and sometimes something else happens.

Close to town a taxi slows down. Cornelius's face appears.

'Hi,' I start. This is a shock.

'Where are you going?' he asks.

Absorbed in my fantasy of him, I'm annoyed that he should disturb it. 'Into town.'

'Do you want a lift?'

The real person is not nearly as magical as the person I was dreaming of. 'Sure, thanks. Come on, Dad.'

We climb in. I suddenly become "out of sorts". Grey destructive clouds grow and twist into ugly shapes. Fantasy and reality rise up for a showdown.

'Come to my email café,' Cornelius suggests cheerfully. He's always smiling. 'It's the cheapest in town. I'll get the taxi to drop us there.'

I follow his lead, Dad hesitates. 'I'll catch up with you in a few days, Alice. I'm going to the Northerner.' He heads in the other direction.

'Bye,' I call after him.

Barely through the door of the café, Cornelius calls out to the Indian girl behind the counter and grabs me.

'Alice, this is Melanie. Melanie, Alice – the woman I've fallen in love with.'

I cringe and smile because I have to. 'Hello.'

I recognise a couple of yachties tapping away in front of the flickering screens. They befriended Dad while Emily and I were away. Now they laugh with Cornelius.

'We'd been convincing Roger that Americans were okay,' they joke. 'That was until you came along.'

They all laugh again. I try to work out what this means.

The scene turns into a grotesque caricature – no one is real. I start screaming inside. I can't stay, I must get away immediately before the outside comes inside me and breaks me into nothing.

I try to sound calm, holding the pieces together, like it's a whim – to pretend, like them. 'Cornelius, I'm going to the market. I'll meet you there a bit later.'

'Sure, I'll be here a while.'

It worked. Cornelius loves email; he taps away on sticky alphabet keys most days.

The market I can cope with; it's straightforward and anonymous, fruit piled up on benches under dark eaves. I am back in the earth. I simply choose a bunch of bananas and hand over a gold coin. Soft yellow pawpaw – three large ones or five small ones? Lettuce and spring onions. Cornelius says spring onions are good for his prostate. I finger the rich red tomatoes and buy a heap. I quieten down in the relaxed swing of the shoppers. I don't need to make any sense of anything until I see Cornelius at the far end of the market, looking for me. It's over. I shrug my grown-up clothes back on and pin them in to fit.

'Come on.' He's impatient. 'My leg hurts, I need to sit down.'

My mind rushes after a different identity. Years ago, I worked in an old folks' home. I take his arm with patient concern.

'Here, sit down. I'll go see how long we have to wait.'

'I hate buses, why don't we take a taxi?'

I'm the one wanting to bus. I could feel guilty. The bus station is noisy and crowded. Buses arrive and leave in belching clouds of filthy diesel. Drivers rev their engines, pretending they're about to go, so the customers will rush on board.

'Why the hell are they doing that?' Cornelius roars.

I stroke his arm. 'It's okay, they're just little boys having fun.'

'Well, they damn well shouldn't be.'

I stay calm and conciliatory. Our bus arrives. The driver keeps revving the engine, even after we're all onboard. Cornelius marches up and asks him to stop.

Fantasie floats against the concrete wall. We swing over lifelines and drop our bundles in the cockpit. Inside is tidy, orderly and clean. The mixed aroma of acrid cleaners and lemon-fresh polish unsettles me, though. Dull shapes in the polished mahogany follow us down.

'Cornelius, your boat's lovely.' I hug my approval. Something is pushing me to get away. I won't let it. I hate it when this happens. My love is twisting into dark shapes. The walls of the saloon shrink, dripping a cold dread. My life is over. I lurch for the companionway to get outside. Anywhere will do, as long as it doesn't have a man in it. I'm vaporising.

'I'm going to the toilet,' I call down in a rush and set off, trembling inside, along the concrete path back to the marina.

Fantasy and reality have crumpled into fear. This is ridiculous. My mind races inside my panic. I can't be accountable. He can't have expectations of me. Solid ground is not solid for me, it keeps morphing. All my possible futures have collapsed into this one here on this boat. I'm inside a nightmare. Cornelius wants to pin me down, trap me, kill me. I'm gasping for breath. Where do these thoughts come from? I don't want them; I want a future with Cornelius. I want to rip my mind out and throw it away. I won't be destroyed like this.

I make my voice steady and light when I return. 'Do you mind if I write for a bit out here before I cook dinner?'

'Sure. I've got a few things to do. A writer needs to write. I understand.'

The focus of my pen calms me down. I can be honest on the page.

"When you open your emails, you'll be taken from me," Cornelius had warned.

He was right. My pen races over the page. My family, friends, old boyfriends have written long warm letters. I belong to them. Cornelius is the stranger. The eons we have known each other count for nothing in the world of time. I was seduced by sex; I don't want to go back there.

Cornelius is flicking through a book and looks up with relief when I reappear. He studies me closely. My eyes are flashing. I'm all seized up, like a frozen rabbit.

'I need to talk. I'm going mad.'

He has no idea the courage this takes.

'Hey, it's okay. You can say anything. What is it?'

He seems uneasy but resilient.

I want to collapse, the mute, and nuzzle my way back into his arms. I need to be bold, I need to change. This is my only chance. I don't know how.

'I want to run away.' I grab some threads of courage. 'I'm trapped. I don't want to hurt you.' I gulp. 'I'm tired of running.' He's listening;

I go on: 'I'm living a recurring dream of being hunted down – I'm always just escaping with my life, always running, nowhere is safe. I've had this dream all my life.'

'Is it to do with me?'

'I don't think so.' He stays calm. 'I'm scared. I don't know who you are.' How can he understand how huge and biting my fear is?

'Where do you want to go?'

'There's nowhere to go.' My voice sinks into a hollow well of despair. 'Will you help me see what's going on?'

He's amazing. 'Sure.'

I keep talking. He listens. Finally my panic drains away.

'Thank you so much. I can't believe how much better I feel.' I move closer, intrigued by his steady confidence. Maybe he does have some answers. 'What gives your life meaning, makes it worthwhile?' I ask, tentatively.

'Mmm, I need to think about that.' He walks over to the navigation table and back. 'Sailing around the world was the best thing I ever did... ' His face lights up, just a little. 'Friendship, being in nature, understanding life in a psychological way, that kind of thing.'

'This isn't the answer I want. Isn't there something deeper? Maybe you don't understand my question?' I sense a problem as he stares back. Self doubt nips my heels. 'Maybe my words don't mean what I think they do?'

'What else could they mean?' He's lost.

'Shall I make a cup of tea? I want one, do you?'

'No thanks. Ah well, if you're having one, okay.'

I escape into the galley, to deal with the crushing sense that ordinary life is totally meaningless. It's all make-believe. I focus on the silver body of the kettle. What do I mean by meaning? Cups, teabags, milk powder. I find everything in tidily-packed-in containers. When the water boils I turn the gas off at the wall. How would I answer a simple question about the meaning of life? English evolved to describe life, not to question its very nature. I stomp back into the saloon.

'Here you are. I've put the honey in.' I sit down with him. 'In some ways we're very different.'

'How do you mean?' He puts the cup on the table to cool.

'Your stories don't take you beyond the obvious and you don't need them to.'

'Thank you, but I'm not sure what you are getting at.'

'I keep trying to live in a world beyond this one.'

'Hey, I'm just an ordinary guy. This is way beyond me.'

'I'm not sure now. Maybe even this other world has been created by my mind. I can never escape my mind which imagines the worlds I live in.'

'I'm sorry, I'm not following you.'

'That's okay. Can I finish? I need to sort this out for myself. Then we can change the subject.'

'Sure.'

I begin tentatively: 'I don't fit in, so I question what life is about, where I belong, who I am.' Cornelius follows up to here then drops out. 'I'm haunted by meaning. Spirituality seemed like an answer, a great escape – now I'm not so sure.'

He doesn't say anything. "She's really crazy," he's thinking.

I return to where I set out: 'I can't get outside a particular point of view and there's nothing absolute about any point of view, not even the spiritual one.' I pause as my mind rushes on. 'What beliefs guide the behaviour of a cell? Maybe you and I don't live different points of view, maybe we just don't know what they are.'

I stop for a second to catch my breath and change direction.

'It's always puzzled me how we live, ignoring the fact that we're going to die. It's very fashionable to talk about the denial of death.' Cornelius nods. 'Maybe it's not denial. Maybe at some level we do understand that we never die, just as we never live in the way we think we do.' I start to get carried away. 'We're part of the endless dance of life that carries us naked beyond the grave and clothed through an ordinary working day. Our cells live and die seamlessly – the passage of life through us. At some level we know we are the intelligence of life living through our bodies.'

I pause. 'There, that's it.'

Cornelius waits to see if I've finished. He claps. 'Well done. You really are a philosopher.' I smile, even though I know he's making fun of me. 'Philosophy was never a strength of mine. I'm more interested in psychology.'

'Come on, let's go to bed.' He gets up threateningly, throws his arm around my waist and tumbles me down. His mouth roams my face, his hands burrow under my clothes, he finally climbs on top of me and we sink down into that mysterious place of love. The night pinks with the colour of dawn and we are still cuddling and talking, relieved and excited to be back in each other's arms. The days that follow are all the same. The morning disappears into the afternoon before we're ready to separate out for the outside world.

I watch fluffy clouds skating across the blue sky, the magnificent panorama of life calling us, as we set out hand in hand down the lane behind the marina. Golden bliss is flooding my body; I'm in love, as happy as can be. The grassy lawn, gravel path, houses, trees, take us down to the beach where we can kick off our jandals to feel the warm sand around our toes and pad down to where it is soft and wet. I stay still so my feet sink under the tide lapping around my ankles. Shiny treasures come in with the tide, little stones and shells rolling back and forth. Thin splashes of white froth land on the sand and dissolve, swallowed up. Cornelius gazes out to the horizon, to a boat sailing away, sails rocking back and forth over the swell.

'When you fall in love, who are you really falling in love with?' he asks suddenly. He stops for a second to pick up a pretty shell. 'I think that maybe it's with yourself.' He smiles at me.

I take the shell. 'That's pretty. It's a little cowrie isn't it?'

'Yes.' The definite affirmative is so reassuring. I return to his question.

'I don't think so. I don't think love is so narcissistic.' We climb back up the beach and wriggle into the shade of floating palm leaves. 'You think we're mesmerized by the delicious feelings of love, caused by a flotilla of endorphins and other chemicals racing through our bodies, creating the "chemistry" between us?'

'Pretty much.' This is Cornelius being philosophical.

I stand up in front of him. 'Okay. I want to look at this in a different way. You stimulate "feel good" chemicals in me. You become the object of my desire, because you make me feel good.'

'Yes, that's what I think.' He's a little impatient now.

'We've been reduced to chemistry. The problem is we don't experience chemistry, we experience love. It's okay – I'm getting there.' I can see he's restless. 'Could the hydrogen atom experience love when it meets its oxygen? Wouldn't it feel relief, even joy as its energy fields restructure themselves around the oxygen?'

Cornelius looks at me like if I've gone mad again. 'I don't know much about chemistry.'

'Both atoms have had to separate themselves, with some difficulty, from their previous liaisons. They hover without the extra electron they need to be stable. They glow and sparkle in their dance around each other and then they come together. It's a transforming experience, shaking them to the very core. Don't you see – chemistry describes the object, love describes the experience. Falling in love is falling for the dance that creates the universe.' I start to prance around in front him. 'It shapes the behaviour of atoms and people and all things in between. Sorry, I'm getting poetical, but this stuff is pretty close to my heart.'

I get serious again. 'Now, I don't want you to think I'm anthropomorphising – I'm not. I'm suggesting that love is a universal phenomenon. Our experience in relationship is essentially the same as that of an atom in relationship. The only difference is that we are conscious of it and can talk about it. That's the only difference.' Cornelius looks pretty doubtful. 'Well, maybe I've gone a bit far, but we humans put ourselves on such a pedestal.'

Cornelius gets up. 'What you say is interesting, I guess. I followed a bit of it. I'm not sure you answered my original question though, about love being narcissistic.'

'Well, I've done enough thinking for today. I'm getting cold – shall we go back.'

'Sure.'

We interlock fingers and set out for home, kicking up sand. I drag him back down to the water's edge to paddle in the warm blue water, clear blue right through to the grains of sand underneath. Bored with the game he pulls me away towards the lane, but I stay barefooted, even on the gravel, so my soles can toughen up. That slows him down, even irritates him. My wet feet are tender and the pieces of stone that burrow in need shaking off, even picking out. I wind my arm around his to speed up, as the cool afternoon jumps off my bare limbs. We swing over the lifelines and back down to our love nest.

21

Cornelius disappears immediately to trim his beard, neat and tidy around his mouth. I poke around for a book and find a small collection in a dark cupboard, floor level, behind some old sheets. They make a little pile on the floor, all dusty and well thumbed, and *Hotel California* by Thoreau is my first choice. Behind the navigation table is a shelf of sailing books, a large fish book, a small fish book, and a book for identifying corals. They look interesting for later.

Cornelius reappears, mortified. 'I must apologise for how I look.' I return the books to the shelves and look up. 'Aging is a terrible process. A few years ago I had my eyelids tucked, on medical insurance. I had some then – I was still working. They hung down over my eyes and I couldn't see properly.' He sits down, drawing his knees together. 'But the rest of me, what can I do about that? I know I'm a mess. I'm so sorry.'

I laugh. 'It's okay – you look fine to me.' I shuffle around in the galley, washing out our cups and putting them back into their cubby holes. I don't tell him that he looks much worse in profile with his saggy chin.

'What shall we have for dinner?' I peer into the fridge at a bit of cheese, a few straggly spring onions and some overripe tomatoes. 'I'll make a vegetable soup.'

I drag out the right-sized saucepan and pick out a couple of onions to slice.

He sneaks up behind me, and right out of the blue I'm belted by a wave of dread, again. In the fairy tale 'Beauty and the Beast', Rose Red turned her beast into a prince by loving him. My princes all turn into beasts when I love them. It's not fair.

I go stiff to keep him away, grabbing the edges of the fridge to get more stable. I grab his arms off me and storm into the saloon to sit down, then I stand up – I can't keep still.

I have to keep him outside me, separate, just a man. I tell myself over and over: the problem is me not him.

I breathe and breathe. I force his image away from me, to get some space. I feel like I'm pushing a concrete wall away from me. I want to run – I need to run away.

I pick up the onion and start slicing. I focus hard on that. With a shaking hand I get out the oil and pour a little into the pot.

'It's okay.' Cornelius puts a hand on my shoulder to reassure me. 'What are you afraid of?'

'I don't know. I was fine a few minutes ago.'

I feel dizzy and confused, like I'm betraying myself by even talking to him.

Slowly I get dinner onto the table – grated cheese sprinkled on top with a little salad on the side. We talk. Nothing gets clear and it doesn't matter. At least I'm talking about it. We turn on the radio to catch up with the international news and then I settle down with my new book. Cornelius rests and flicks through an old sailing magazine. Mainly he rests.

Next morning I'm scared and ready to run again, except the only place to run to is Dad's boat and that doesn't seem much of a choice. I open some more Orere plum jam for our toast. Cornelius is suitably impressed, except he worries about his weight. He hands up strong coffee which steams a rich aroma into the cool air. We sit outside in the morning sun. The boat is moving, ever so gently and all the masts in the marina wave delicately together.

I creep into the shade of the dodger. 'I need to sort this horrible stuff out. I'm so panicky.'

My voice is deadpan except for a deep shaking rumble, a sense of impending annihilation – me as nothing. "I can't need people, it's too risky," I'm thinking.

I shake free of my discomfort, focusing outside of me: stainless cleats and shackles, neatly coiled rope, the dodger with its seams starting to unravel, light creating shadows everywhere I look.

Cornelius listens but he doesn't say much.

'I don't understand who you are. Maybe it's because you're American?' Cornelius's smile seems a bit enigmatic. I let his silence slide. 'I've done lots of work on emotional issues in meditation, but for some reason it hasn't fixed this. I don't know why.'

Cornelius looks up, curious. 'I didn't know you looked at emotional issues in meditation.'

I recover my equilibrium and slurp the last dregs of coffee. 'I was involved in an experimental wing of Tibetan Buddhism. My teacher was Wongchuk, a Canadian Rinpoche. He was a bit like you actually – larger than life.'

Cornelius perks up even more at the comparison.

'He worked with Tibetan spiritual traditions, Western psychotherapy, Western mystery traditions. He used art and movement – anything to free us from our unconscious patterns, the prisons of our conditioning. Got into lots of trouble with the traditional Tibetan lamas.' Cornelius spreads a thick layer of jam onto some more toast and licks his fingers delicately. 'Actually, all the work I've done looking at my issues has been through meditation. I never did counselling.'

'Why not? It seems like it would have been very useful.'

'I never had the money and I was skeptical about the depth of the work. In meditation I got into some pretty subtle and terrifying places, but the instruction was always to just observe. That's all that is required to take us to liberation. That's what we were taught.' I stop to prepare my toast. The jam is both tart and sweet, rich in colour and taste. 'What about your therapy?'

Cornelius becomes thoughtful and intimate. 'Well, I started in group therapy. It was very confrontational.' He hesitates before going on. 'I wasn't popular and it took a long time for me to accept that I was the problem. I had a pretty dysfunctional personality. Then I went into personal therapy. My therapist loved me. Maybe that was the most important outcome – being loved.' He pauses to think, then lets the thought go. 'That's enough talking. Time for a rest.'

I collect the dishes and lick the jam off the knife.

Cornelius used to play flamenco guitar. As a young man he studied in Spain for two years, plucking, picking and strumming the fire in his belly into music. His fingers are still fine, like a musician's, even though he's pulled on sheets and halyards for twenty years now. Gypsy music fills the boat. I sink into the melody and snuggle against his chest.

'Cornelius, there's something in this music I recognise.' I listen more deeply. 'I know what it is: there's Islamic chanting, inside it.'

'You could be right.'

'I wonder what the roots of flamenco are?'

'I don't know.'

Cornelius doesn't know what to do with my endless theorising.

Evening falls, the fluorescent light spreads a wan lemon light over us. We undress and snuggle up in the saloon, kissing and stroking.

'I don't suppose you've ever had to deal with this before?' Cornelius suddenly spits, almost mocking the situation. He pokes his droopy penis.

I recoil from his pain and mumble. 'No, it's a new problem for me.' I look up through the hatch into a dark sky pinpricked with silver.

'There's nothing worse than being excited, seeing you under me, wet and impatient, and then looking down to discover my penis is fast asleep.'

I swallow him up in my arms. 'You're the best lover I've ever had. You're incredible in bed. This doesn't matter.' It doesn't.

'Maybe not to you,' he tenses up to be angry, then sinks back into forlorn, 'but it does to me. I don't think I can stand not satisfying you.'

I cup his chin in my hands, turning his face to mine. 'I love you.' My kiss fills him up with all the tenderness I can find.

'You know … ' He drags himself up to sitting, happier now. 'I haven't told you this because I didn't know what to make of it.'

Yes?' I re-curl myself into his arms.

'I was sailing down to Vuda Point from Savusavu – it must have been a week before you arrived with your Dad.' He pauses to glug down the glass of water on the table. 'A small flying fish leapt out of the water as high as the spreaders. You've seen them – they're about twenty feet above the water. It was being chased by a larger fish.' His hands spread out two feet. 'They arced over the boat together through the spreaders and then fell back into the sea on the other side.' He takes in a long slow breath. 'How likely is that to happen?' He beams at me while I shake my head. 'It's almost impossible. I think it was an omen. You are quite some woman, you know.'

Morning sun floods the companionway. Eyes soft in a mist of spent passion, sarong tight around my waist, I run fingers through my hair and wonder if I look okay. The perfume of ripe pawpaws and pineapple is sweet and voluptuous.

Cornelius spins around from where he's pottering at the navigation table. 'I've been thinking about Max.'

My eyes stop on the bowl of ripe fruit in the galley. His hands on my shoulders force me to pay attention. My heart leaps. He looks straight into my eyes. Max has come up in several conversations. I've been very honest about how caught we were in each other.

'I need to say something. This is my final statement about the dilemma you two are for me.'

I freeze. A faint smell of diesel wafts in from outside – a large yacht motoring towards the exit crosses our bow. The smell of fear comes from my body.

'I have no option but to love Max,' he says.

'What! I don't understand.' The engine sound becomes muffled, then all is quiet.

'Max is probably a neat guy. You obviously love each other. There must be a lot of Max in you after ten years. You even told me that I'm like him.' He keeps staring me straight in the eyes. 'Given my love for you, the only way I can be free of this conflict is to love him as well.'

He pauses then, to let my thumping heart settle. My mind is racing in all directions at once; it can't make any sense of what he's saying. 'You're free to make your own choice when the time comes. That's all I have to say.'

My mind finds a focus, it suddenly remembers The Water Babies, a story I read many times to my children for the understanding I needed. All the men in my life are the faces of the one man I have called forth as woman. The penny drops. I get it. There has only ever been one man in my life. The past is in the present, same shaping. Cornelius and Max are the same man for me! Cornelius knows all of this. He is my teacher. He is amazing.

Cornelius busies himself with the radio, to wind down from his magnanimous gesture. Morning slips into afternoon, shadows grow from the trees outside and creep across the pocked concrete to our boat.

'We need to get out. Let's go to the estuary,' I plead.

I wait for him in the cockpit, looking across the jumble of steel wires, masts, mooring lines and hulls hugging the concrete rim of the marina. Vuda Point is Cornelius's favourite place in the world. Some boaties use this cyclone hole as a toilet. I use the toilets on shore. He would like to buy land close by and settle, visiting yachties for company, hens running free, growing old. There is no one in America for him but his old mother, one daughter and two grandchildren. His daughter only allows him to stay three nights. He's been gone too long to return now. He wouldn't fit and he certainly wouldn't be captain of his own boat.

He looms up large in the companionway. Walking is good for his back, at least he thinks it is, but he's unsure about the dog-like feeling he gets when I suggest it. Maybe he should bark! His strides are large and strong. I work hard to keep up. We sweep behind the marina, striding past low-roofed Indian homes with their small gardens. The country smells in the fresh air fill our lungs. I take his hand.

'I've been thinking,' I start.

'That's dangerous,' he laughs.

'We're so caught up in our fears at the moment. From the outside it must look pretty self indulgent. I mean, why don't we just get on with it?'

'Psychology is interesting. Fear limits our lives and gets in the way of happiness.'

'That's right.' I jump with a shout. 'I want to be happy, I just don't know how.'

'That's what it looks like to me.'

I tug at his arm. 'Slow down a bit, I can't keep up.'

He stops. 'Let's sit down. Then you can think better and I can listen properly.'

We sit under a large tree on the side of the road. 'I want to know who I am underneath all my fear.'

'You sound a bit like my shrink,' Cornelius answers in the pause. 'He used to talk about being authentic and real. I think you're right.'

'I'm always dancing around in images of myself, trying them on to see if they fit, re-assuring myself I exist. If I knew who I was I wouldn't need to do this – I could be myself. I'm not and I can't stand it.'

He brushes a strand of hair from my face. 'It's okay. What you're doing is important, I can see that. You do want to sort your shit out. I hope you do. Maybe then we'll have a future.'

He picks up a stone and throws it at another stone on the road. 'The fucked-up ideas from my mother almost destroyed me. Without psychotherapy I wouldn't be here, I know that.' He takes my hand and stands up. 'You think too much. Come on, let's go down to the water.'

I turn away, perplexed, confused. 'The strange thing is ...'

Cornelius puts his hand over my mouth to stop me. 'That's enough.'

At the bridge, the tide roars under us. Silvery tummies flash past. Their flailing fins and tails are powerless against the sweeping current. Bigger fish coast the edge, eyeing their next meal. Some lucky sprats will soon get a chance to turn into something much bigger. I climb down the side of the bridge to look. A fishing boat stuck in the mud starts to float and little mangrove seedlings brace themselves for a gentle wash.

Dusk is falling as we return. Houses start lighting up, flocks of birds speed home to their bamboo beds in a noisy clamouring, dirty old cars speed past, spraying dust.

Cornelius roars after them, 'Damn them! What are they doing here? Why don't they slow down?' I stay as still as the sinking light, trying not to react to his outburst.

We're seated at a plastic table with metal legs, under shade from a striped umbrella, on a concrete pavement more stone than cement sloping to the street – having lunch, café style, in Lautoka. I bite into dark sticky chocolate cake and Cornelius forks noodles and chicken in under his moustache. The coffee is Nescafe but strong enough, with lots of milk and sugar. Old cars and taxis slide past, almost at a walking pace. Pedestrians, mainly Indian, straggle over and line up for fatty chicken, cassava and noodles. The elephant trunks of soaring palms stand over the traffic down the road, and the hot, hot sun keeps everyone slow. Children dash from shade to shade across the street.

'Hey, Steve,' Cornelius calls. He whispers across the table, under tortoiseshell Raybans, 'He has a large catamaran. He's on his own with inherited money.' A lean well-groomed young man ambles over. 'How are you, Steve? This is Alice, the woman I'm madly in love with. How's your cat?'

I accept the compliment more easily now and smile without the grimace. Cornelius puffs up to hide his discomfort, and outstrip his imagination.

They swap a couple of sailing stories and then Steve ambles on. We recognise a few other boaties, hidden behind sunhats and glasses, heading towards the general store for supplies.

That same afternoon, we wrap up together in the saloon for a late afternoon nap. The air, a teasing mix of warm and cool ruffles my skin. The outside world sways ever so slightly in the companionway. Weedy flowers in a small jar are starting to wilt. I must remember to give them water. A couple of my T-shirts are almost on the floor – must remember to pick them up as well.

Cornelius stretches his arm up the wall. 'This is not going to work. If I can't make love to you, I'll lose you. One of those young men out there will ask you out. He'll have a hard cock and you won't be able to resist.'

Our bodies stay glued together, in perfect repose, utterly happy, drinking their full.

'I'm not interested in any of those young men,' I shout, to shut him up.

'Not now, maybe, but wait and see.' His eyes roam around inside himself, gripped by the thought.

'You'll destroy us with your delusions, do you know that?' I sit up to shake him. 'Stop this. This is dangerous.'

'You're right.' He becomes bashful, embarrassed, and then playful. 'When I was sailing with Ursula I often became paranoid, not about men – she never looked at another man. She never looked at me either, but that's another story. She used to calm me down.'

'Well, I'll do my best.' I climb onto his chest and tickle him. 'Why can't you think rationally? It's easy.'

'Wait, I want to show you something.' He pulls away to sit up, then clambers over the life-raft box wedged in between the mast bulkhead and the side of the sofa. From the cupboard opposite he retrieves a folder, from which he produces the evidence: the scientific confirmation and therefore the justification.

'Look at this – it's an aptitude test. I paid $500 for it. I did well in everything except reasoning. I find it hard to be rational.'

I scan the document. 'Boy that's some justification. I've read that difficult emotions hijack reason. Someone who can't reason under pressure is dangerous.'

He doesn't answer, but quickly returns the folder to the back of the cupboard.

Stretched out in bed that night I wonder about the younger man. I don't know the future. Cornelius rolls over and starts snoring. I lie awake for hours, mulling things over. Day breaks and I snuggle around him, aching with love. He finally rolls over and his mouth covers me in kisses. We tumble together, limbs snaking, feet twirling, linked together like chainmail. How dare the night separate us! How dare our nightmares come between us! After the dark night full of dark thoughts, we burrow our way back together, gasping for redemption.

'Minds make trouble for hearts. Our hearts aren't confused,' I whisper.

Cornelius leaves me to compose myself and sit up for the cup of steaming fresh coffee he produces. A fine bliss is rippling through my body, rippling out into the boat and beyond. All I feel is this bliss. I'm glowing with love – goddess and child all mixed up in a woman's body.

We sit outside in the cool morning to have breakfast and greet the day.

'Why don't you move onto my boat? You're here most of the time and your father wants a woman for his boat.' Cornelius passes some toast and strokes the hair on his chin.

'Do you think I should?' I jump up and twirl around a couple of times. 'What a scary idea. I haven't lived with a man for thirteen years. I'd be waking up in your arms every morning. Mmm … I wonder what that would be like.'

He follows my sarong around. 'You're my dream come true. Do you know that? I've wanted you on my boat from the moment I saw you.'

I shiver with panic and excitement.

Dad arrived at the marina yesterday. I find him pottering and listening to the BBC.

'Hi, Dad. I'm moving onto *Fantasie*. I've come to get a few things.' I wait for a reaction. Dad's right leg, crossed over the left, shudders and jerks a little. He turns down the radio. 'Cornelius would be horrified though if I lugged across my bike and tent and panniers and pack and piles of clothes and books.'

'Sure, they're fine here. I'll get out of your way.'

'How are you getting on with your advert?' I put on the kettle.

'I've had a few replies, but I'm getting cold feet. What would a sailing companion expect? I don't want something I can't get out of.'

I break into a broken twitter of a laugh. 'Dad, that's the story of your life … and mine too.'

'I'm a bit caught. You and Cornelius should sail together if you want to go around Cape Horn. You need to learn about his boat.'

I could have done more to look after him. I crumple up inside. I clean up the galley. We're not good on the boat together when we're not sailing. I nose around for a few things. When we set out, he had romance on his mind just like me. Guilt is love gone rotten. It has a bad smell I can't get rid of.

'Why don't we all go sailing somewhere. You could come on Cornelius's boat. I'm tired of hanging around doing nothing. I'll ask Cornelius.'

I sink down into the comfortable clutter of a half packet of coconut biscuits on the table, marmalade lid growing stinking cigarette stubs, smelly clothes left where he took them off. I relax into the floral upholstery, under tapes and books falling down the shelves behind me.

'That's a good idea. *Dream-maker* would be safe here. You haven't seen the Yasawas. They're over-rated, but everyone goes there.'

'I'll come back and let you know.'

I bundle up my clothes and creams and peck him on the cheek. 'See you soon.'

22

Back on Cornelius's boat, I unpack my things into their new homes. 'A man,' I say quietly to myself. 'We're a couple now.' The word 'couple' catches in my mouth. We have to look out for each other. I arrange my oils and creams on the small shelf above the toothpaste-splattered sink in the toilet. His possessiveness is endearing and flattering now, but the novelty won't last. I glance in the mirror. I don't trust this romantic fantasy.

I carefully fold my T-shirts in the corner of a poky cupboard, up against the fibreglass hull. What happens when the ordinary wakes me up in a drifting boat and I turn to a man I don't want to know? I fold my sarongs and undies on top of the T-shirts. I think of all the stances I've taken – too busy, over-excited, anxious, passionate, fearful, angry – all ways to escape the simple burden of loving a man, as a man, not as a portal to my beloved.

Cornelius watches. I lay colourful sarongs on the settee to lift somber green and mahogany tones. He smiles awkwardly at my taste. I arrange odd flowers from around the marina in a jar on the table. He's seeing ahead into brown petals on the clean floor, jar tipped over and water lifting the mahogany veneer.

I spray rose water infused with essential oils into the air, to herald my arrival as 'woman.' I play with us lightheartedly, as if fantasy can protect me from the dread of annihilation. I spin around in his adoration as if this can make me exist, so that when I slow down I won't fade away.

I reassure him; 'I'm not going to rearrange your whole boat. I've made too many homes in the last few years. Also, I'm not good at cleaning. Making a place look pretty is my limit for now.'

I hug him proudly. He seems disappointed – I'm not sure why. Through my new homemaker eyes, *Fantasie* is cluttered and disorderly. Two toolboxes face me stubbornly on the floor of the small galley and on the bench above mountains of plastic containers stack three and four high. Fishing rods collect dust around our bed and an old tarpaulin covers outside odds and ends that have ended up inside. I hadn't noticed until now.

'A glass of wine,' I declare and pass the bottle and corkscrew.

I'd prefer to go out, but Cornelius likes it here. He doesn't want to be reminded of bars. He doesn't need them now. We're a couple: each other's cuddle rug. Cornelius works on the fridge, I write – harmonious, domestic, threateningly comfortable. It doesn't seem real, it couldn't be real. I'm dressing up in someone else's clothes. It's what I want. I'll stay here until someone finds out. I'll dream under the soft light, melting into Elton John's love songs for as long as I can. We're going to make love tonight and sail the high seas tomorrow. This is the best dream I ever dared dream.

The Yasawas are a small group of islands to the north, on the west coast of Fiji. *Fantasie* glides effortlessly into the swell. She changes from a lovers' nest into a sleek water animal.

'Cornelius, she's beautiful. The sea creature under our feet has woken up. This is what she was built to do.'

I rush to pull up the main. I want to sail. Dad steers, so that Cornelius can show me how. *Fantasie* speeds up until she's leaping through the waves, ripping apart the sky, taming the wind to our will. A bold sun fires down. My muscles pop and scream against the wind as it whips the headsail out. I need every ounce of bulging flesh to winch it in. Dad helps. I switch on the electronics and confront Cornelius with my diagnosis.

'We're sailing in a five knot wind just forward of the beam and we're doing six and a half knots. Isn't that impossible?'

He smiles, 'Yeh, well, she's a racing boat.'

I leap onto deck, into the wind that's everywhere – belting waves into rugged mountain ranges, ripping the headsail out into a huge belly shuddering against its sheets, sweeping my hair to the heavens. I've never felt so alive.

Naviti Island looms up. Coconut palms grow from colouring-up shadows of land.

'We'll go in here Roger, for the night,' Cornelius says. 'Alice, you can furl the headsail now!' – his voice is commanding.

I leap into the cockpit. Dad helps. Together we roll up the sail, till it's all quiet. I take down the main by myself, Dad keeping the folds inside the lazy jacks. I drop the anchor and then we shrink away inside for dinner and conversation. Life has scarpered, just like that. Conversation ricochets between Cornelius and Dad, well rehearsed positions and points of views taking turns. There's no one talking. I collect the plates and dump them in the sink and creep outside into light falling into the dark of the brooding ocean.

Cornelius pokes his head out of the companionway. 'You're a real minimalist when it comes to social chatter.'

'I'm sorry. I need to be alone, that's all. You and Dad have lots to talk about.'

He shakes his head and disappears, then pokes back up. 'Can I get you anything?'

'No, I'm fine thanks.'

My breath frees up, my belly relaxes. Lumps of land move jerkily with the boat, the sea sighing, twinkling with the moonlight. Bites of noise and light filter up the companionway. I soften into giving myself up – to the land, the sea, the night sky. I melt away again from my human faces.

Cornelius calls me back: 'Come on down. It's getting late.'

In the morning we motor around to where the beautiful manta rays swim, and drop anchor. The sun plays peek-a-boo with clouds shadowing the broken water grey.

Dad rows, while Cornelius and I swim in search of the graceful 'sea angels'. We snorkel back and forth across the opening where the narrow bay turns out to meet the sea. We surface together. I splutter, mouthing the snorkel out of the way.

'Where will they be? Where it's shallow or deep?'

Waves splash into my mouth. Dad plays with the oars and water in the way he might have done in Raglan harbour, where he was a young boy growing up. Cornelius shakes his face free of the lumpy water. He'd rather be in the dinghy or better still lying down in *Fantasie*.

'I don't know. I haven't been here before. Did you see the sharks?'

'Yes,' I shout across the rushing hush of the sea. 'They looked quite big.'

'They're much deeper than you realise. They're huge.'

'Should I be scared?'

'They're not the little reef shark.'

'Mmm … that's exciting.'

I won't be scared. A group is still patrolling, way down below. If I don't look at them, I'll be fine.

'Only sharks,' I finally call bravely to Dad after we've crossed over and over and further out. We clamber over the soft walls of the dinghy and he rows us back to *Fantasie*.

'It's your birthday!' I suddenly remember, 'You're seventy-eight today. Happy birthday!'

Cornelius holds onto the toe-rail while I hang the painter correctly over its cleat.

'Congratulations, Roger. If I'm still sailing at seventy-eight, I'll be very happy. You've done well. What do you put your youthfulness down to?'

Dad plants himself solidly on the wobbly floor of the dinghy and grabs the toe-rail as well, just in case. 'Well, to be serious, I think exercise is the most important thing, and being positive.' He stows the oars under the seat. 'Women and whiskey are important as well.' He turns back to Cornelius. 'A positive attitude is what really counts.' I cringe, because I know what's coming. 'My advice is to do what you want to do, not what society tells you to do. The world is your oyster.' He pauses and climbs up onto the side of the dinghy, a little stiff and bow-legged. 'I didn't start living until I was fifty. Then I took a year off work and went sailing. When I was your age, Cornelius, why … I was in my prime.'

He smiles at Cornelius in a way I don't understand. Cornelius isn't exactly a man in his prime. Is Dad making a statement or just remembering the good old days? He certainly looks good. Cornelius doesn't reply. His smile is inscrutable, his white teeth perfectly silent.

I discover a packet of instant chocolate cake mix in a food cupboard. 'I'll make a birthday cake.'

I'm not sure how old that is,' Cornelius warns.

I add extra baking powder – I'm not sure how old that is either. When the surface of the cake bounces back under my finger, I take it out.

Cornelius looks it over. 'It hasn't risen at all.'

'I know, but it'll taste good.'

Cornelius and Dad settle into their stories, like two old salts. They talk for hours about batteries, radios, wind vanes, anchors, charts, weather, rigging, sea maps, the adventures they've had. I waft in the background with cups of tea and food, relieved that they're getting on so well, pleased not to have to join in. When Cornelius rests, Dad reads.

'Roger, I'm sorry to keep lying down – the pain in my back is much worse when I sit. I feel like an old cripple, but what else can I do?'

Dad's face shifts between grimacing and good cheer. 'Some exercise might help, although I've read that rest is good for backs.' He doesn't approve of Cornelius's degenerating body, not when I'm planning to sail around Cape Horn with it.

'You're so like each other.' I hand them each a cold beer and sit down. 'You've both chosen a life of sailing, you're both romantics and you both like talking.'

Then I spring up like jack-in-the-box. 'I need to get out – I'm going snorkelling.'

Cornelius turns to me, wondering if he's done something wrong. 'Try my blow-up kayak, it's tied on deck.' Maybe he's meant to come.

'Okay, I'll give it a go.'

I force myself, but I'm tired. I need to be on my own again. I've never been happier. I have more than I could ever have dared wish for. Slapping at the waves, I paddle the kayak over to some rocks at the harbour entrance and drop over the side. I'm inside a bubble that's grown too big. Something's wrong. I need to get out before it pops.

This whole sailing adventure isn't real. Why isn't it real? This is what I had planned – to grow a new life, inside a new bubble. What about my life in New Zealand, my children? The elastic is stretching, taut and ripping. I'm too far away. Nothing much to see in the water. My arms are tired, but I row on and on until there's nothing to do but turn back, now heading into the wind, towards *Fantasie*. Tears well up, maybe from the wind. The gentle breeze carries the scent of the land. I miss her softness. I miss who I was before I met Cornelius.

The memories help tie me back together, keep me strong enough to re-enter the galley and slice fresh barracuda into fresh herbs and coconut cream. We caught the fish on a trawling lure on the way over. Dad killed it by pouring vodka into its gills – an instant, pain free death. He showed me how to scrape the scales and lift off the fillets. I slurp down a glass of wine, ready for any conversation. Dad starts expounding his metaphysical world view, but he knows to be careful – the lioness in the galley will pounce.

'I firmly believe that you create your own reality. Alice, you would agree with that, wouldn't you?'

I thump the knife down on the bench, to assume my position.

'Dad, it completely depends on what you mean by *you*. Are you trying to tell me that you created this boat and the ocean and Cornelius and me?'

Dad isn't listening. He's singing his song, mixing the melodies to suit the occasion. I mark time with my interjections.

'This is one of many possible worlds. I've always been interested in the power of the mind. If you believe in suffering, like Alice here, then you will suffer.' He turns to Cornelius, to make sure he is following. 'Suffering is an illusion. I refuse to be pessimistic. I have never understood the pessimism of Buddhists. Every morning I wake up into a wonderful world. Life is a precious gift.'

I get wound up, on cue. 'Dad, that's not fair!' I shout. 'The Buddha teaches a way out of suffering. How can you say you've never suffered?'

I stalk back into the galley, to find the salt and chop an onion. I'm tired of this conversation. I'm tired of getting so worked up. We haven't changed much over the years. My claws uncurl. My tail thrashes the air. I wait.

Cornelius, well trained in the art of conversation, is determined to be interested, but he can't make sense of our intellectual extravagance.

'What is this talk of creating your own reality and suffering being an idea rather than a basic inevitability of life? I'm a bit out of my depth.' He turns to Dad. 'Roger, are you and Alice disagreeing about anything real? Maybe this argument is only about whether the glass of water is half full or half empty.'

I smile and leave Dad to wriggle with that one.

'Dinner's ready. Dad, another glass of wine?' I hold up the bottle. 'Cornelius, can you fold down the table?'

I lay out our birthday feast: marinated fish, rice, a fresh salad and rock-solid chocolate cake for dessert.

'Roger, to your good health.'

Our glasses clink.

I congratulate him. 'Like an unpinned Catherine wheel, you spun out at a tangent to the conventional, sparks flying wildly.' I sip my wine. Dad's shoulders jerk with pleasure. 'At fifty, you broke the school rules and slipped from the straightjacket of social conscience.' I start singing: 'Those were the days, my friend. We thought they'd never end…' I sit close to him.

'Remember when I visited you at your bach by the sea. There were precious books in your bookcase: *The Autobiography of a Yogi*, *The Autobiography of a Western Yogi*, *In Search of the Miraculous* and others. Remember?' Dad nods. "I think you'd enjoy reading these", you said. I followed you into the spiritual tide.'

He glows in my appreciation. 'As a child, you crossed a watery tide by horse to go to school. You went to war and struggled for an education afterwards. You've had quite a life.' I turn away, trembling with sudden emotion. I suddenly realise we had different agendas in our spiritual searching. I was looking for love, but Dad was looking for freedom.

Dad turns to Cornelius. 'Life is an adventure and you can have any adventure you choose. When you've had all the adventures you can dream up here, you go to the next plane for more. I believe in other planes of existence, so when I die I will wake up in one.'

He's warming up, his rosy cheeks glowing.

'I know what you mean, Roger. I certainly chose a life of sailing and I did dream of meeting someone like Alice.' He tries to tie down the free flow.

'That's right. The more unlimited your thinking the more unlimited your life.'

I distribute more food. 'New-agey' people like Dad aren't interested in truth, they just want more fun, more power, more freedom to play with more new toys. Sometimes I find it hard to keep the difference between Dad and me clear.

Cornelius swallows a mouthful of rock-solid cake. 'I'm interested in behaviour, not ideas. Behaviour describes who we are, not ideas. My life is about sailing and friends. I'm that straightforward.' He tells us a short story from Hollywood.

I retreat to make coffee and formulate my answer. I place the steaming cups in front of them.

'I believe that the idea came before the behaviour – not necessarily a conscious idea. A genetic idea drives a fish upstream to look for food.' Dad and Cornelius start at my aggressive, pontifical manner. 'Ideas drive desire and behaviour. Faulty ideas, like the ones I have around relationships, lead to self-destructive behaviour. Good ideas increase happiness; bad ideas increase suffering. The idea comes first – it names reality from a point of view. Without a point from which to view, nothing exists, action is not possible.'

Dad doesn't waste a breath. 'I couldn't agree with you more,' he bursts out. 'Ideas create the reality we live in. I keep saying this. Because you hold onto the idea of suffering, Alice, you will suffer. Why can't you see this?'

Dad just doesn't remember yesterday's loneliness. He didn't grow up swimming in it. His mother loved him. I remember her. She was a big protective woman with long silvery hair and blotchy liver spots on broad hands that dug the garden and held us close when we stayed in the weekends. When we sucked lead pencils, she washed the poison out our mouths. She cared.

23

Cornelius remains an enigma. A week ago, when an old acquaintance of his passed his boat, he spewed vindictive rage after him, within hearing! Why didn't I describe this incident when it happened? Because I was ashamed. I know the instinct of shame. I shouldn't be associated with him. Whenever his mother comes into the conversation, he tenses up, curls his lip and turns his eyes hard and mean. This morning a wine bottle rolled out of a cupboard onto the mahogany floor, making a small dent.

'Who didn't put the wine bottle away properly,' he roared. 'Look what it's done to the floor!' He waved his arms, burst red, and blew out into a full-blown tantrum. 'This is my home!'

Dad and I watched. We didn't say anything to each other.

In the afternoon I was struggling with the winch to bring in the headsail.

'What's wrong with you?' A shockwave clapped me from behind. 'Don't you know how to sail? You're too slow!' He raised up, tall as the heavens – Zeus smashing thunderbolts together. Dad rushed across the cockpit to help. Afterwards Cornelius wasn't embarrassed. He acted like nothing had happened. To me everything had happened – my whole world had come tumbling down.

I try to understand. He was abandoned by his father as a young boy and brought up as an only child by his sociopathic mother (his words). She turned him into a powerful alpha male, for herself – forget about him. Maybe the pain in his back is about his mother? Sometimes he seems like a caged animal ripping itself to pieces on the bars.

The boat rocks gently, the tide slips past swinging us slowly towards shore. Shadows of coconut palms run together up into the hills. Why can't Dad see how real this suffering is? I never understood why the Buddha declared his first noble truth to be the truth of suffering. I thought it was pretty obvious. Even running after pleasure is a kind of suffering isn't it? I dress my life in glamorous clothes, mystical interpretations, grand questions of meaning, and Dad has his 'created realities' and 'boundless freedoms'. Maybe we are the same as Cornelius. Maybe we're all only running after pleasure and away from pain, maybe we're all only suffering.

Dad and Cornelius huddle over *Fantasie*'s radio, which isn't working properly. Dad was a radio technician during the war. Cornelius's radio isn't quite as old as Dad's, but it doesn't go any better. Every now and then a squeak or hiss or garbled voice, caught by the box, spits up the companionway.

I gaze over the water. I didn't understand most of what my teachers said in the early days. Their teachings seemed trivial or overly complicated. Nonetheless, I sat in respectful awe at their Birkenstocked feet – bare toes poking out in summer, calf-length socks keeping them warm in winter. I chanted exotic Sanskrit words, soaking up the dark maroon mystery of it all. I didn't have a clue. I thought powerful meditation experience led to liberation, whatever liberation was.

One day Wongchuk said, 'Know the wholesome for the wholesome and the unwholesome for the unwholesome.'

I had scribbled this down on my pad, unsure of what wholesome meant. We were all scared to ask questions because sometimes he had a go at us.

He said, 'When you know for yourselves that certain things are unwholesome and bad, then give them up. When you know for yourselves that certain things are wholesome and good, then accept them and follow them. If you can do that,' he had paused, covering the class with a majestic sweep and beaming smile, 'you will awaken in this lifetime.'

Obviously I had missed something, because that seemed a very easy thing to do. I mull the teaching over. If the Buddha meant 'ideas' when he said 'things', then I can see now that liberation is a long way from where I am. I don't know the ideas driving my crazy behaviour, polarising my life. Cornelius doesn't even have a clue that his behaviour is crazy, let alone the ideas driving him. How can we give up things we don't even know?

"Exactly," I can hear my teacher say. "This is the work of liberation."

Something needs to be done. 'I'll shinny up the mast,' I announce. *Fantasie* doesn't have any mast steps and someone needs to look out for coral. Let it be me! I lock my hands around two halyards and pull up with everything I've got, legs clamped around the mast to stop me slipping down, to rest and to help push up a little. My biceps grow like baby sandcastles. Can I do it? Seventeen feet of mast rise up above me, to shinny up and up, pulling on the halyards, to the first spreaders. Pride keeps me straining and struggling, not letting go for anything, until I just clamp my hand over the metal cross piece. I almost can't do any more. I start to freeze. I can't, I can't give up. I haul myself over, shaking uncontrollably, becoming a rag doll. No, I can't collapse now, I have to get to sitting. My breath shudders to a stop and I gasp at some air. My legs almost collapse under me as I stagger to vertical, hugging the mast. I'm terrified to look down. Breathing, chest heaving, shaking, breath slowing down. I wobble, the hero – wire arms tight around the mast now – on lookout for coral. I don't know where we're heading; I didn't look at the chart. 'No wonder you end up ship-wrecked all the time', a little voice inside me quips.

Cornelius calls up, 'Which way should I go?'

'Where are we going?' I yell back, pointing to shallow turquoise water. 'There's coral over here and there.'

He shouts back impatiently, 'I don't want to know where the coral is, I want to know which way to go.'

We're surrounded by bommies, their coral heads lying just under the surface of the water. I can see the difficulties. I just don't know where to go from here.

I call as loudly as my shaky voice can, 'Do you want to go up the coast or into a harbour?'

He's nonplussed. 'What's all this about?'

The confidence in his voice thrills me. Behind the wheel, he knows who he is. He calls again, 'Just one more thing.'

I turn around.

'I want you to get divorced so you can marry me!'

I wobble and hold onto the mast ever more tightly. I blink and blink, knocked off my perch. I'm suddenly terrified and excited. I suddenly see everyone at our wedding, looking at myself through their eyes, winning, losing, approval, disapproval, success, failure. Every pair of eyes sees me differently. There would be a lot of Alices getting married. I'm not sure any of them is me. I don't know who I am or what I want.

From up here I can see a long way, a grand panorama – islands stretching out in all directions, with harbours and safe channels, coral reefs, fluffy clouds and blue boundless sky. I become furiously angry. What's wrong? Why can't I live my life here? I want to kick and scream and raze the heavens. I want to destroy it all. Why? I stare and stare, demanding an answer – there must be one. I look down on Cornelius and Dad from on high, into the petty world they inhabit. I will wait forever if need be for the answer to come.

It arrives.

I can't stand the miserable imperfection of being human. That's it! That's all it is. I cling ever more tightly to the mast. I can't accept my fall from perfection, from grace, from the whole, and the fall of everyone around me. I won't put on the clothes of a dirty, grasping, suffering human life. I won't accept the intolerable mediocrity of being human.

I look down at Cornelius. I'm an impostor, playing with his love in a make-believe world. Sadness swoops through me, a softening, an accountability. Is this why we never became real? Neither of us could stand the imperfection of a miserable human life, so we drowned in our love. I spin slowly on the spreader and look down at the deck blazing in the sun. We have been defeated by our shame, the shame in the difference between what we wanted from life and what we got and the distortions and pretences that grew to make it seem okay. This shame is our unacceptable fall from perfection into

time and it is there festering in all our secrets and dissatisfactions
and fantasies. It is our suffering.

A seabird soars high above, wings spread to the heavens. Birds
find their way safely across vast oceans. An inner compass, a body
reckoning, steers them home, wherever home is, whatever it is
– if that's where I'm even going. Home is beyond suffering, the
destination of the spiritual journey. Like the bird, there must be
something in my bones that knows where I'm heading. I have to
trust that. There are no charts for sale, showing the way through
my reflections and confusions. I won't find an old timer's sketch
of reality, marked with Xs, under Dad's navigation table. Faith is
the mast I'm clinging to now. I drag this difficult word out, like
an anchor from a musty bottom locker. I don't even know what it
means.

I come back to my actual position, standing on a spreader up in the
heavens, holding onto the mast for my life. I crouch down and hang
my legs over the spreader, then stomach and finally chest. I let go the
mast and grasp the halyards. Feet walking down the mast, I slip back
down to the deck. The vanity that got me up there turned out to be
pretty useless. It didn't have a clue what to do once I was there.

We sail around the island, looking for shelter. Waves, broken by
wind, turn back on themselves, reflecting off the land. Smooth clear
faces momentarily point one way only to collapse and reform in the
opposite direction.

Dad takes the helm. Cornelius helps me with the main, until I
have it safely lowered inside the lazy jacks. I cleat off the halyard and
tighten the mainsheet to hold the boom steady. We motor into a quiet
harbour, made up of two islands joined by a ridge of sand. A large
yacht tried to sail over the ridge a few years ago, I guess because it
wasn't marked on a chart. The wind is blowing onshore so we're on a
lee shore but there's nowhere else to go. We inch in as close to shore
and as far out of the wind as we can get.

'Okay, drop the anchor,' Cornelius calls.

Dad helps me feed out the chain, hand over hand as it rattles out of the chain locker and over the roller – under control – down into sand or coral, we aren't sure which.

'Sixty feet should do it,' Cornelius calls.

'Can you put on the snub?' he asks as I come back down to the cockpit. 'It's in the locker.'

A snub is a piece of rope with a hook on the end. I hang over the pulpit at the front of the boat and swing the hook into the chain, a couple of times before it catches, then tie the loose end to a cleat on deck. By letting the anchor chain out a little more, it starts to hang loose between the ends of the snub, so the anchor pulls on the cleated snub rather than the windlass. Rope has some give, so the boat swings more gently and it's quieter. The windlass could, theoretically, turn or be damaged in a strong wind if the anchor was pulling on it.

Dad watches and whispers encouragement while I attend to this task.

'Alice, I'm sorry to have to say this, but if it came to a choice between looking after you or the boat, I think Cornelius would choose his boat.' He takes a step back, to leave space for my reaction.

I jerk up as predicted. 'What! What a strange thing to say. Of course he would look after me!' I quickly recollect some incidents. 'I don't know, maybe not.'

I walk away, dismissing further consideration, back to the cockpit, the astringent taste of imperfection still in my mouth.

Cornelius joins us with a glass of wine, attentive and funny.

'Next time, make sure you look at the chart before you scamper up the mast. Roger explained the problem. By the way, we'll be here another day. The wind's against us and I'm not sailing back to Lautoka in a head wind.'

'That's fine. I'd like to go ashore tomorrow,' I reply.

The sun slips down through the cool, condensing sky. The 'creamy milk' we were continues to curdle. My mouth sours with the part I'm playing – 'succumbing to flattery' and 'being sexy' – curds of self disgust. I'm running away from myself and as my chin sinks into my fist, a heavy resolve gathers.

'Cornelius, come here and sit down.' I look out to sea, not at him. 'I don't want to be an object for you to claim, admire, possess, fondle, comment on. I'm not a thing.' I almost trip over the spit in my words. 'I want to be your friend. Friendship is different from this.'

Cornelius looks at me seriously, until I face him. He likes these discussions. 'Hey, we *are* friends. What am I meant to do? You're everything I want in a woman. I can't keep my hands off you.' He stops to re-curl a sheet that's come loose. 'Don't you like that I find you so attractive? It won't always be like that. You'll get old, so enjoy it.' His eyes flash mischievously.

Rigging clatters and tinkles in the growing silence. I stare at rust stains dripped from the stainless fittings into the fibreglass. The swell rocks us ever so gently.

Last night Dad held the floor, topped up with rum and coke. He declared: 'Men are driven primarily by their sex drive.' He should know, he was a natural science lecturer.

'Women are the real motivation behind everything we do. Power, money, fame and sailing mean nothing without a woman. They're all ways into the beds of beautiful women. Don't you agree, Cornelius?' Cornelius wasn't sure of a diplomatic response and Dad didn't wait for one. 'Ask any of the men on boats here if they aren't thinking about women all the time. They're happy if they have a woman and miserable if they don't.'

'I've read that men think about sex on average every six minutes,' Cornelius finally responded.

I turn back to Cornelius. 'Is what Dad said last night true? Do you see me mainly as a sex object?'

Cornelius believes in being honest. 'Certainly that's what men are primarily interested in – the shape of your bum, your hair, your face, your body – anything else is a bonus.'

Heat rushes to my face at his cool answer. I never understood this about men. I look at him. He's so sure of himself. I always thought, or was it that I pretended, that men liked me for my mind. We sit in the falling light; wind swings us slowly toward shore; the cool breeze caresses my arms and cheeks. The evening is idyllic, this whole sailing trip is idyllic. I gulp wine, my insides in disarray.

Cornelius leaves to see if Dad wants some company.

'Hey, Roger, did I tell you about the time I almost lost my boat way up in Alaska … ?'

In bed, under a damp duvet half covering us, shadows of fishing rods in the corners, dark grey peeping down the hatch, I start again. I used to pretend the pain away. I can't anymore.

'I need to talk about a couple more things.' I can almost see his eyes.

'Sure, what is it?'

I almost can't talk. It would be easier to clam up and forget. No, it wouldn't be anymore. It's huge for me to be talking like this to a man.

'What keeps couples in relationships?' I sit up, then lie down, then sit up again. 'What do they want beyond the desire for a mate and wanting life to be easier and not wanting to be alone?'

He doesn't say anything. They seem good enough reasons to him. What's my problem? He rolls over slightly to face me in the dark.

My voice rises to angry despair: 'And what's the price? What's the compromise? Do I have to pretend to be happy?'

Surely I've said too much. I can't help it. 'I'm lost,' I plead. 'I'm not saying we're over. I'm frightened.'

Shadows grow darker around us. He doesn't have an answer and I'm not expecting one. I'm frightened to stay and frightened to go.

I stare past the shadow of the toilet and sink into the solid door that separates us from Dad and the rest of the boat.

Finally he holds me close and whispers in my ear. 'I love you, but you're always free to follow your own dreams. It's your choice whether you stay or go.'

I roll away, still angry. How can his life be so straightforward? I knot my brow to help, staring into the dark mahogany-panelled door. My questions will never have answers. They never have. My jaw clenches with frustration.

Cornelius scoops me back in his arms. I unroll like a soft white maggot and burrow into his warm flesh. I find his mouth and kill my brain with his kisses. We fall over and under each other, like the sighing, whispering sea. None of my problems makes any sense anymore. We make love and fall away into the dark night. I sleep safely in his arms, his woman, and wake under the spell of a searching mouth and tongue.

24

I'm under the dodger, fixing my dilemmas into my journal, hidden from the sun that would evaporate us all. A local Fijian with his son and daughter putter out from the island in a long boat.

'Cornelius, come up here. We have visitors.'

The father holds up an empty jerry can. 'Do you have any petrol?'

Cornelius and I look at each other.

He answers quickly, 'We need some water and have some laundry. We've a little petrol to spare, not much.'

The man smiles in agreement.

'I'll go in with them,' I quickly offer.

Dad and Cornelius prefer to stay behind.

Simple houses hug a communal sandy yard, swept into arches and squares inside clipped twiggy shrubs around the edges. Large mango and breadfruit trees provide shade. Houses, some bamboo, some fibrolite and iron, spread out along sandy lanes. Women and children gather around. It seems so familiar, so natural, like a human curl in my genes.

I fill water bottles under the village tap and leave our washing with Johnny's wife.

'Would Aime like to come back with me for a visit?'

Cornelius warned me that women on boats miss other women and plants. I miss children.

I help Aime over the lifelines, holding her hand. 'Come downstairs, I'll show you around.'

She follows me down the companionway.

'This is the toilet and our bed. The table folds down like this.' She nods shyly, peering into the corners, following my gestures. 'There are food cupboards behind these squabs, and this is the radio we use at sea.' I don't know how much she understands. 'Would you like some tea and toast?'

She nods politely. I fold down the table in the cockpit, sit her down and leave to attend to the food. Cornelius and Dad stay pretty much out of the way. Ridiculously excited, I ignore her request for my watch and look away when she slips her hand into Cornelius's pocket looking for change. Pretty curls frame her pale face. She sits across from me in a broad smile and a dusty pink dress, picking at her food. She would rather go inside and find treasure in the cupboards.

When Cornelius motors us ashore to pick up our washing, the women invite me into one of the huts.

I point to some writing on the wall, in Fijian. 'What does that say?'

'It's from the Bible,' a younger woman replies.

'Do you have a translation?'

Cross-legged on the flax matted floor, I read out loud from an English Bible: *Enter ye in at the strait gate: for wide is the gate, and broad is the way, that leadeth to destruction, and many there be who go in there: Because strait is the gate, and narrow is the way, which leadeth unto life, and few there be who find it.* Matthew 7:13-14.

I put the Bible down reverently, grateful to be here. I miss spiritual teaching and community.

The women each bring out shells for me to buy, ones they've gathered off the beach. When Cornelius appears, they lead us down a shell path bordered with shrubs and flowers, past more houses to the home of the chieftainess. We offer kava and she welcomes us to the village. I ask permission to walk over the island. She asks for money and clothes. This village has a lot of visitors, so they have the right to our charity, she says.

'Alice, are you finished there?' Cornelius pokes his nose into the open thatch hut where I am looking at more shells. 'Let's go for a walk.'

'Sure.'

'I don't like the village,' he declares.

We walk along the beach and talk as we used to, ruffling golden-white sand with our toes, gazing into clear blue water, stopping in the shade of the coconut palms, looking into perfection.

'I've been pondering your question about meaning,' he starts. 'For me, meaning is this walking along the beach together, this happiness, this exquisite serendipity. I'm living a life I've chosen, one I fought for, not the life my mother or society wanted for me, but my own. It's enough.'

I motor us back out to *Fantasie*. Cornelius teaches me to swing the dinghy in a big circle and bring it up close, facing the right way, stopping the motor as we gently bump the hull, perfectly placed, perfectly timed. I try it a couple of times. A great sweep of wake follows us round, sweeping us into the boat. As the pattern becomes predictably familiar, I fine-tune my approach.

When Dad appears to take the painter, I pass him my shells to admire.

'Ah, conch shells and a pretty cowrie. They're very nice.'

'Remember those beautiful shells you brought home from the islands years ago? You used to dive for them. These are ordinary by comparison.'

'Ah, yes. That was a long time ago now.'

Two young fishermen in a long boat pull up alongside and ask if we would like to buy some lobsters.

'Sure. Tonight I'll cook my special lobster dinner,' Cornelius brags. He turns back to the fisherman. 'Do you have three?'

I shriek, 'Cornelius, look, at the two turtles! One is probably a hundred years old.'

The fishermen see our distress. 'It's okay, we're not going to kill them.'

"You're lying," I want to shout. I stare at the overturned bodies, heads lying on one side, limbs flapping uselessly. My stomach turns. Nothing I can say will save them. When they leave, Cornelius goes on and on about how terrible it is. I can't see the point. It might make him feel better. Dad is philosophical – he's seen it all before.

I sit sadly while Cornelius breaks open the carapace of a freshly boiled lobster and folds out its flesh.

'Does anyone want to go for a swim?'

'I'll come with you, Alice,' Dad replies. 'Cornelius, what about you?'

'No, I need to look after the boat.'

We head for the small reef at the entrance. Cool water washes me free of our harsh air world. I become a water baby again, splashing and swimming, bubbling like a fish, following the jewel-like flickering bodies around the coral. What freedom! Nobody to care. Nobody to comment.

'Dad, you can row back to the boat when you like. I'll swim back for the exercise.'

I fall into the steady rolling rhythm of my body, now a sleek, powerful sea lion. The sea caresses me. This is how I was before Cornelius came along – I was carefree, I didn't have to be anyone else's dream, I was safely wrapped in pearls of seaweed from my beloved. This is how I was before the grownups came along and took me away. I imagine that I'm swimming in this perfect world.

I swim back to *Fantasie* and haul my carcass into the dinghy, wobbling across its sagging belly to where I can grab the lifelines of the mother ship and clamber aboard. Cornelius is hoisting the sun shower.

'Here, let me soap your back.'

His lips follow the soap until I'm squirming with delight. He passes a towel. He follows my smell, my bottom, my smile. I rub the towel through my hair. I've fallen for his dream of me, haven't I? Naked in the setting sun, I dry my arms and legs. I'm pretty happy. My legs bristle red. I'm fooling myself? I slip down the companionway to hunt for clothes.

Morning wakes me gently into his expectant gaze – he's impatient for the night to be gone. His unbridled passion sweeps me up. He throws me down on the bed and climbs on top of me, tender and violent both. I scramble away and reach out for him. I draw him down onto me. I keep disappearing, tossed away into deep dark space, lost from myself. Waves and waves of powerful energy rush up through my surrendered body – uncontrollable and unstoppable, on and on – until I am far too far away, obliterated. Cornelius notices the wild distressed look in my eyes.

'It's okay,' he reassures. 'You're safe here.'

I coil and uncoil, I can't stop the energy rushing in. It's happened before, but not this full on. The power of the universe is infinite. How much can I allow in before it destroys me? My voltage regulator certainly isn't working. I drag myself to the corner of the bed, against the hull, to where I'm safe from his hands and mouth, a small furry animal ball. I'll hide in the darkness until I come back. He brings me a cup of warm sugary tea. I wait and wait, but I can't find my body. I tie on a sarong and pull a T-shirt over my head. My fingers push through the knots in my hair as I step gingerly down to the floor. I don't know what's become of my mind or what's happened to my body – I don't recognise them. I can pretend to be normal.

'Good morning, Dad,' I croak, looking away, creeping past into the galley. Shakily and excruciatingly self-conscious, I make us all toast and coffee. Cornelius and Dad pretend that I'm normal. I prop a book in front of me and pretend to read. I close my eyes and let my mind sink, so it will gather the pieces of me, bundle them up and return me to myself. Nope. Wispy cloud in boundless space is all I feel. This has happened too many times, this love making, blowing me to smithereens. I'm finding it harder to remake myself afterwards. My eyes look out from places I don't know. Sometimes I seem to have the eyes of a cat or a rock or the eyes of dark space? The shape of my mind is no longer clear.

'Alice, are you ready to go ashore?' Dad asks. 'I need to stretch my legs.'

'I'll stay on board, Roger.' Cornelius still doesn't like stretching his.

I row, willing strength into arms I can hardly feel. Ashore, trudging through the soft sand, I can't make anything solid – I move in a blown-out faded world. Friendly faces arrive to show us around. I smile vacantly, and follow Dad's lead, glancing through open doorways and across weedy gardens, registering in a dull way the detail of these lives.

'Can we walk up into the hills?' I ask the woman next to me.

'Yes, certainly. The children will take you.'

I take off my sandals so my toes can wriggle in soil and stones. Dad relaxes and chats in bits and pieces. He's happy to be finally onshore. Excited children rush ahead and back, taking our hands, telling us their lives in broken bits of English. I'd much rather be alone. I help with words like banana, pawpaw, breadfruit tree. The bush is open and rough. I crave time alone to walk over her body in me. Cornelius objectifies me; the children objectify the trees for a game. It's a deadly game, this separating out – turning into curds and whey rather than staying as sweet creamy milk. It's the evolutionary game of becoming self-conscious, of naming a world to live in, of creating our realities.

As we return to the boat I formulate my next way out of the game.

'I want to go ashore and be on my own for a while. Over there,' I point, 'where there are no houses or people. Can I take the dinghy?'

Cornelius accepts my request.

'It's too rocky to drag the dinghy up on shore. I'll drop you off and pick you up. Do you want to go now?'

'Yes.'

We motor across the bay to where I can step out into warm, shallow water.

'Can I have an hour and a half? It'll be getting dark by then. I'll meet you back here.'

'Sure, enjoy your walk.'

He motors away.

I start out slowly, tentatively. I hesitate like a bashful young girl facing her awkward young lad. I'm alone on the land. My eyes peer through the scrub and down the beach. Time trickles like precious drops of water. I gasp. She is so beautiful. My heart leaps out in all directions and buries itself in the leaves, shells, stones, in every pattern and movement. I am returning. I find myself snuggled up inside all the delicate creatures of life. Deep peaceful eyes look back at me – my eyes. I gaze through rocky footholds to myself. I'm held in a sacred spell, in the radiance of an intensely gentle, all-pervading love.

I walk up and down the beach and off into the scrubby bush that falls down to the rocks, disappearing inside everything I look at – melted, utterly at peace, lost to myself. I stop to pick up the odd pretty shell and turn over a leaf; I listen to the muddy stream trickling into the sand, the sea lapping at the shore. The stony sand scrunches under my feet, the sounds, the touch, telling me about myself before I was taken away to a human world. I am made of this fine beauty, but I can't hold on to it – it trickles through my fingers like grains of sand. I look out to sea. *Fantasie* rides peacefully at anchor.

Part of me will accept the human journey, part of me is still angry. I turn a shell in my hand. Mystery turns in the spirals, we share calcium bones. What happened? I never stop long enough to enter the touch of a broken stone or whirl with a falling leaf. I keep forgetting myself. Do Dad and Cornelius have any idea what happened? Tears well up and trickle down my cheeks. We've reduce nature to an attractive backdrop. We are her children. She grew us. I stare sadly into space and look at my shell in the sand. Society says that if we own things we will be happy. I laugh a little inside. Maybe ownership is a way of trying to come back together. The more things I own, the bigger I get.

The sun glows on the horizon. A bowed human shape appears on *Fantasie* and climbs into the waiting dinghy. The motor starts. I enter the tide to wait. As he arrives, the sun slips away and the sea turns a dark shadowy velvet. How can I tell him where I've been? I draw curtains behind me and climb into the dinghy. He waits to hear my story, ferryman between worlds, eyes still blasting hostility towards the locals. He charges them with slyly lying and manipulating, out to get what they can. He's still holding onto the lives of the turtles we saw dying yesterday. The hostility is his own. It doesn't belong to locals or turtles.

'I had a wonderful time. Thanks for picking me up.'

My hand settles on his knee, he turns the boat around.

'How's Dad?'

We're on our way again. I grab Cornelius's arm. 'I'll go up again on lookout for coral, but first come here.' I drag him to the navigation table. 'I don't want to look stupid again.'

I take the chart outside to match it with the coastline, turning it around so that the layouts fit. 'Women always do that,' Cornelius laughs.

Then I haul myself up, more easily this time, and still burst with pride when I get to standing and call some good directions down. When the coral reefs have slipped behind, I slide back down, and in my hurry trip over the folded main and large winch, then half stride, half fly into the cockpit for my next job.

'Pull up the main,' Cornelius directs.

Dad keeps the battens inside the lazy jacks while I winch it up, careful not to over-stretch the leach. I cleat off the halyard so the rope runs the same way under the turns and follow Dad back to the cockpit for our next job.

'Now you can both unfurl the headsail. Roger, you take the furling line. Alice, you winch in the sheet.'

I get confused about which way to coil the sheet into the teeth of the winch. Dad comes to my rescue.

Cornelius watches us spring into position. I stand with my feet planted solidly in the cockpit so I can get enough purchase and turn the winch without stopping, until I'm on fire.

'That's right, you're doing well.'

Dad tells me to stop when there's the right amount of belly in the sail for the wind. I'm still learning. Cornelius is bossy with Dad, but Dad does what he says – he's crew like me.

'Can I steer?' I ask when the cockpit's tidy and I've curled the windward-side unused lines neatly around the winches, the way Cornelius taught me, and I've put the winch handle away.

'Steer for that point of land,' he directs.

Focused and steady at the wheel, I can't stay still. How can I? I'm full of a passion for living, I want to rush with my body into the hugeness of life, to fly to the heavens and back, but I can't, I'm stuck here. Life is magnificent, how can I not want to throw myself wildly into her arms, how can I not want to break open into the wind all around and be carried away. I can't do anything with her.

'Dad, can you take the wheel? I'll go make us a cup of tea and fix a meal.'

Cornelius looks into the wind and back to the tell-tales, pieces of cotton on the sail. They're drooping a little – they should be horizontal. He pulls in the sheet, just a little, automatically.

A squally wind rises in the night, swinging the boat round and around, snaring the anchor chain in the coral. Heavy coils drag back and forth, rasping and scraping.

Cornelius rolls over, with the duvet. 'The anchor chain was re-galvanised in Fiji. It's being ruined.'

Neither of us can sleep. I fret: 'We put out more than a hundred feet of rope. What if it slices through on the coral? How deep is it here? We're wrecking the coral.'

'I don't think I put out too much.' Cornelius rolls over again.

'Couldn't most of the chain be on the ground? It seems risky to me.'

We lie awake listening to the noise for far too long.

Cornelius capitulates. 'Let's go and pull some up. I'm not sure how much I put out now.'

It's close to midnight, but Dad's still reading, all alone. This is not his boat, which is good and bad.

'Dad, I'm making cocoa. Do you want some?'

I wouldn't but for him. I'm too tired. We chat until the smeared cocoa paste has dried out around the bottom of our cups.

By early morning, the wind has turned even further around and we don't want to tack home, so we're here for another day. Dad and I need to stretch our legs.

'Alice,' Dad starts, as we bob away in the dinghy, 'Cornelius may not be up to sailing around Cape Horn. He's old. I have real misgivings.' He looks down as if this conversation is his unpleasant responsibility. 'His boat is run down. It would take a year of full-time work and thousands of dollars to get it up to scratch.'

I listen, but I don't care. I answer like a child. 'I do want to sail with him. He loves me. He's had a lot of experience and he knows his boat.'

Dad has always been overprotective. Doesn't he realises that I never stop to cross the 't's or dot the 'i's? I just go and throw myself away.

We carry the dinghy up above the high tide mark and drop it on the golden sand. I follow behind him, my dad, salty streaked, crumpled T-shirt and loose walking shorts, white head bobbing. After half an hour through the bush he's had enough.

'I'm going back to sit on the beach in the sun.'

'Sure, I'll be back in a couple of hours.'

He watches me disappear through the long grass whipping at my legs. A good track leads under the trees to where it's dark and damp. Young banana palms and cassava sticks grow in small plots, cleared to let the sunlight through. Vines run rampant over the trees. A man carrying a grass basket full of kumara tubers passes. I don't see any houses. The centre of the island is an upthrust phallus of solidified volcanic fire. I stroke ferns and seedlings growing from footholds in its rock.

I reappear on the beach at the appointed hour, light as a barefoot wood nymph. Wings crumpling in the heat, I fold them at Dad's feet. They quiver as he chats with the locals. A young man turns to me. I smile some more – I can't help it – and I tell him about the green forest and black rock. My voice is light with the beauty and wonder of the day. On an empty beach far away from anything of consequence, I fill to overflowing with outrageous pleasure. Looking out on the bluest sea, an extraordinary blue, this infinitely precious moment suddenly becomes painful, because none of it belongs to me – I can't do anything with it. I am nothing and everything. Kneeling silently in the golden sand, I stare into crystal beauty, brilliantly-alive space.

We row back out to *Fantasie* as we rowed in, father and daughter adrift in the universe, stubby rubber-nosed boat parting the breeze and sea through to infinity. That we should exist at all is impossible. That we should be bobbing through the waves like this is ridiculously significant and nothing at all.

Cornelius has baked fresh bread. He's prepared the barracuda for another meal. We scramble down into the saloon. I grab cold beers from the bottom of the fridge and open a can of New Zealand butter. We gather around the warm bread and slice big hunks.

Dad starts, 'Cornelius. I'm worried about my boat. It's time we went home.'

He's finished his book.

Cornelius looks directly at him and scowls. 'You know I don't like sailing to a schedule. I'd rather wait for a good wind.' He looks at Dad's set face. 'We can have a go tomorrow, if you like.'

I slice more bread.

'Thanks. I do want to get back. We've been away six days, which is a long time to leave my boat.'

Cornelius glares at me. 'Tonight I'm having a valium.'

'Sure, wrap your arms around a pillow. I'll be fine.'

In the cool evening I sit alone in the cockpit writing my journal, as I do most evenings. My pen traces unintelligible scrawls over the page: "Will I be left as anything more than a spent firecracker – ragged black cardboard, red at the edges, dampening in the morning dew?" I jump to the next page. "Sexual bliss isn't pure and soft like mystical bliss or cool and fine like the bliss of clarity – it's thick and sticky."

I start again: "Impressions, intimations, ebb and flow through my body like the tide. Maybe this is the passion of life before it finds a human voice."

I gaze out blankly into the dark. 'Life' – what a word. Four little letters. My pen races across the page again.

"Thought is our human measure. It can't bring to order the unruly mix swirling in my breast. It can't beat into submission the wild running sea. Thought can't sort Dad and Cornelius and me into tidy boxes and keep us there." My pounding heart drives the pen. "Back behind this screaming is another place, the cool clarity of pure awareness, behind my humanness, behind all the measuring and weighing that started with my birth.

"I'm like a dogged emerald-winged fly trying to climb a slippery glass tumbler. I stumble, fall, pick myself up, push against, hold on – to what?" My pen spills a glob of ink, but it still rushes on. "Dream! How many dreams have I dared dream? This glass tumbler is the work of dream. This magnificent dream of sailing – I hold onto it as if this were the only place I can surrender to life. I dream of sailing the seas as if they were mine and I am its mystery. I was born to dream and I don't know why. I'm haunted by not knowing. I keep slipping down the slippery walls into the sticky bliss. I don't understand the nature of glass. One day it will break into a thousand pieces. Then I will be free of my dreams. Is this what the Buddha meant when he talked about waking up into reality?"

I remember sitting in front of Wongchuk, starry-eyed, quivering with excitement. I had pushed my way as far to the front of the large group as I could, eager for a spiritual suntan.

His voice boomed around the room, his eyes wide and intense.

'The first noble truth the Buddha expounded to the few disciples who gathered around him at Sarnath was the truth that suffering exists.'

That took me aback. "You have to be joking!" I thought back then. "What kind of great truth is that?"

'The second noble truth he expounded was that suffering has a cause.'

My teacher's voice carried weight and authority. I was almost impressed. I wasn't – I was incredulous. That suffering has a cause seemed so obvious it was lame. I shuffled uncomfortably on my seat and looked around the hall of spellbound students.

'The third noble truth is that there is an end to suffering,' Wongchuk continued.

I couldn't figure how he got to that from the first two truths. He wasn't a logician, that's for sure.

'And the fourth noble truth is that there is a way to the end of suffering.'

This was starting to sound like a word game now. I was bored.

With that, the teacher asked for questions and, as there were none, he got up and left the hall.

There it was, in a nutshell, the greatest teachings of the Buddha.

I didn't even bother to consider them, they seemed so banal. I wanted a much richer food to dig my curly-pronged fork into. There is suffering. It has a cause. There is an end to suffering. There is a way to the end of suffering. These were the four insights of the Buddha that liberated him from suffering. Maybe I should look more closely at his teachings.

25

We return to the tranquility of Vuda Point with its necklace of seedpods snared in rope, protected from the wind. Dad gathers his things and I stroll with him around to *Dream-maker*.

'Now you can rest and do things in your own way.' I hug him briefly.

'Yes, it'll be good to be on my own for a day or two. I'll see you later.' He unlocks the boards clamped across the companionway and disappears inside.

Cornelius puts on some music, ten discs at a time – soulful guitar tunes, lilting melodies warbling passionate despair. We weave our love back into a thick cuddle-rug.

Two days later a knock on the hull swings me out of Cornelius's arms.

'It's Dad.' We've hardly pokes our noses up.

'Hi, do you want some coffee? I'm just about to make some.'

'Sure, thanks. Hi, Cornelius, how are you?' He sits down stiffly with his calendar. 'This is going to come as a shock. To keep to our plans, we need to leave for Vanuatu on the third of August. That's only a week away.'

He passes me the calendar.

'Alice, you'll have to sail with me. So there it is.' He drains his coffee mug. 'I'll be off now to let you sort things out.'

Cornelius and I reverberate in the shock waves.

'He was going to find crew so I could sail with you.'

'For some reason he's changed his mind.'

'I have to sail with him.'

'That's okay. I know.'

I lay out cutlery and plates, standing the knives and forks straight up and down, evenly, plate in between – focusing on the detail, to hold us steady. Cornelius will have to look for crew. He may have to leave after Dad and me.

I bring the food to the table, one plate at a time, and set it down with more care than usual, shaking inside.

'This is scary,' I admit.

'We'll be okay. Your responsibility is clear.'

'Anything could happen.' I dish the rice first. 'Why did Dad change his mind? He doesn't want me to sail with you. I'll see him tomorrow.'

We eat in silence.

When I meet Dad next morning he is puffing away, a lot on his mind.

'Why are you wanting to leave all of a sudden? You'd been planning to stay indefinitely.'

He stubs out his cigarette. 'I wouldn't let you sail anywhere with Cornelius. His boat is unsafe.' He looks straight at me. 'It certainly wouldn't get through a category one inspection in New Zealand.'

He lights another cigarette.

'What do you mean?' I try to stay calm.

'All his equipment is falling apart or broken. It's quite inadequate.'

I'd noticed some raggy sheets. 'What equipment?'

'His radio. The hull needs a good paint, and where are all the photos and personal things you would expect to find on a boat that was someone's home?'

'What have these things got to do with anything?'

'There're fishing lines hanging all round your bed and no shelves in the galley, just stacks of plastic containers. These things tell me a lot about who he is.' He stops for a couple more puffs on his cigarette. 'He's overweight, carrying around big globs of fat; he's a shipwrecked sailor. I don't want you sailing anywhere with him. He doesn't even know how to sail properly.' Dad is shaking now, ejecting the cigarette smoke like a dragon, not himself at all. 'Look at his life – he left a good career in Hollywood in his early forties. That's far too young. He threw away his life. How could you take him seriously?'

He snorts involuntarily.

I've never heard Dad talk like this about anyone. I can't make out what he's actually saying.

'Well, Dad, maybe that's what you think. I love him. I've never been so happy.'

I make us a cup of coffee and change to the practical matters of getting ready to leave – shopping, moving back onto his boat.

I heard myself in Dad's voice, but I'd locked the spiteful voice away where it couldn't hurt anyone. How much should I reveal?

I walk slowly around the concrete perimeter and back to *Fantasie*. I will tell him everything, otherwise the secret will poison us.

'Hi, how did you get on?' His fingers stroke his prickly chin as his eyes dart inside and out again.

'Let's sit down. It's serious. It's only what Dad thinks, it's not what I think, okay?' A heavy pain glazes his eyes as I repeat the conversation. 'Why do you think he turned on you like this?' I keep my knee against his thigh.

'Well, he doesn't trust Americans. He doesn't like us.'

'He doesn't think you're good enough for me. He's worried about my safety.' I pause. 'These are ordinary things. I've never seen him so desperate.'

We look for clues. I jump up. 'There's something I want to read to you.'

I hunt among my piles of clothes and books and creams. 'This may be the answer. I wrote it earlier this year.' I enunciate my words, American style, clearly and slowly: 'People are talking about themselves when they talk to you. People can't betray you, they can only betray themselves.' I put the journal down. 'This is the key.'

Cornelius doesn't follow, but he's listening.

'When Dad was talking he wouldn't see you as a person. He didn't acknowledge any similarity between you both. You're the same in lots of ways. You're both getting old and you both have old boats.'

Cornelius starts to remonstrate.

'I know yours is a cool racing boat. There's no comparison between *Dream-maker* and *Fantasie*; nevertheless, they're both old.' He relaxes again. 'You both abandoned careers to go sailing. Dad's equipment is always breaking. I re-glued blades on his wind generator three times. His oven doesn't work and his new outboard doesn't go properly. I could go on and on.' I jump up and down with excitement now. 'Don't you see, he won't respect your life, the choices you've made. He refuses to accept the life you have chosen.'

I wriggle around. I'm not expressing myself very clearly. 'There's a subtlety in here that's hard to express, to understand even. It's to do with the way we destroy other people by judging them instead of respecting their choices. I do it and I try not to. I do it to pretend I'm something I'm not, that's it, to believe I'm not the same as you, that we're not all in the same boat. Dad can't accept you … '

I pause as a tidal wave starts to overwhelm me. I'm now working hard to hold back tears so I can finish, and my voice hardens to stop the shaking now taking over my body.

I speak quickly, all in a rush to get it out. 'Dad is saying this about himself. He can't accept the 'shipwrecked sailor' in himself. He can't accept that his life has come to this. You represent what he can't stand to see in himself. You are an unacceptable affront to the fantasy he has about himself.'

The lonely despair in Dad's face is all I see. Cornelius waits for me to calm down. He faces me, hands firm and reassuring on my knees.

'There's something I noticed about Roger. He never talks about his feelings.'

'Yes, I wonder if he knows what he's feeling. That's why he goes on and on about not suffering. He tends to disappear into fantasy, happy ever after, like me.'

'What's wrong with fantasy? We all fantasise. I fantasise about you all the time.'

'No one is real. I should know, I've struggled with fantasy all my life. I know what it does. Other people are only the portions I need for my fantasy – faces in my mirror. That's all I see. No one is real, no one exists independently of me, no one exists in their own right. Fantasy is an act of hatred against the world, it's a self-imprisoning bubble.

Cornelius shakes his head and looks around the saloon and then back to me. 'What on earth do you mean by real? I'm totally confused.' He would pull his hair out if he had any left. He stalks up and down the saloon now. He helped create the fantasy of Hollywood movies – thin, conveniently whitewashed storylines that reduced characters to two dimensions.

'That's a very interesting question,' I reply.

'You're not making much sense. I like fantasising and thinking and dreaming. This is what makes my life rich. It makes me happy.'

'My question is – do you have a choice? I think you disappear into fantasy to escape, without even noticing you've gone. You turn me into a fantasy because you couldn't stand to live with me as a real person.'

'Do I love you or my fantasy of you?' He pauses. 'Maybe you're right. I'm not sure I would like you without the fantasy.'

'There you are! How destructive is that?' Cornelius looks totally dismayed. 'Don't worry. I'm saying this about myself as well.'

'You win.' Cornelius interjects. 'That's enough. We're in love, so let's enjoy it. Come over here.' He drags me across to him, takes me in his arms. 'How can you say this isn't real?'

I wriggle from his arms, light the stove and open a fresh carton of milk. Cornelius doesn't eat biscuits – they're fattening – but I do. 'I'll put on some music.'

'Sure.'

'Do you want a cracker and cheese?'

I rattle about in the kitchen, hunting for food.

Wisps of smoke from burning sugar cane stubble curl into the still, blue sky. Myriad masts wobble in the water. I walk the concrete perimeter swinging a bucket of dirty clothes, murmuring 'hello' to a fellow yachtie trundling his load of groceries. A marmalade cat springs across my path to chase a bird that has just landed on the grass after chirping sporadically from a scraggly tree a minute ago. A couple of Indian tradesmen measure squabs for new covers in the cockpit of a nice-looking sloop. The wife flicks through coloured offcuts in the sun.

In the laundry I dump my bucket under the taps and sprinkle in powder, then twist my arm back and forth vigorously, hand stiffly spread like an agitator – a human washing machine. Once I've rinsed soap bubbles off everything, I wring the clothes as tightly as I can into damp sea cucumbers. The laundry is usually full of chatty women offloading washing for the marina wash-maid to do. Today, I'm alone.

Clean washing swinging in my bucket, I set out again. Locals, repairing and repainting boats parked up on the hard, turn my way. 'Bula,' they wave, smiling from lean, hard-muscled bodies. There's no law stopping them working me into their fantasies. Back on *Fantasie* I hang my panties and bras bravely into the wind.

The day is as beautiful as it gets, fresh and warm. The galley bursts with bowls of fruit and vegetables. Light melodies dance around us. Cornelius starts roaming in an undirected way, which means he's hungry.

'What's for lunch?' he grizzles from low down in his stomach.

I spring up. 'I'll make us some toasted sandwiches.'

We have bunches of fresh coriander and spring onions, tomatoes, onions.

Before I know it, I'm right in the middle of a 'missing my kids' episode. I keep chopping through a downpour of tears, and hunt for cheese in the bottom of the fridge. I want the tears to go away. I drag the frying pan from under a stack of pots and pour in some oil. I hardly know what I'm doing, I'm so de-arranged. I want to smash everything in this stupid boat.

Cornelius looks up. 'Are you okay?'

'Yeh, I'm just missing my kids.'

The sandwiches slide into the bubbling oil. The oil spits nastily back at me. 'Do you want some cold water?' I ask him. We have a container in the fridge with limes in it.

'Sure, thanks.'

'Let's eat outside in the fresh air. Then we can go for a long walk.'

I fill our cups with cold lime water.

Sandals, sunglasses, sunhat, a spot of sunscreen on my nose, I'm ready to go. Cornelius copies me. 'Let's go to Saweni Bay,' I suggest.

'That's five kilometres away at least.'

'Is it that far? Well, we have all afternoon. I'm leaving in a few days – maybe I'll never come back.' I tug his arm impatiently.

We walk steadily, without talking. Birds sit in a row on the power line, snuggling and preening each other. Long slow trains, both full and empty of sugar cane, rumble past. The fields have no cane left. Staked cattle eat the hard stumps left behind and new leaves sprout through dark soil.

Thin black Indian children with shining teeth play ball on the street and laugh to us as we pass. Cornelius approaches, his hand outstretched. 'Give me five.'

The low-roofed, arched Indian houses are familiar – we've walked this road many times. A sign appears: "Ices for sale." I tug Cornelius's arm. 'Let's go in and have one.'

Everything shifts slightly. Flowers, breadfruit trees, hazy blue sea in the distance, all fill with light. I become empty of my thoughts, the weight of gravity – nothing but radiant light. We are walking in pure crystalline beauty, just like that. It's easy now for my mind to switch.

Saweni Bay is gentle and quiet, nothing special – a golden beach, lazily beautiful. Several yachts shelter from the vagaries of sea and wind. Young men throw themselves into the water to cool off. There is no hurry, no one is important and there is no problem. We sit on the sand for a bit, then set out back the way we came. I move quickly to keep up with Cornelius's large, loping strides.

Back on the same bridge, we watch schools of small fish leap through the air, holding onto their lives for now. Again, every glance is dissolving into beauty, into light, and then the image is as if it never was. I no longer exist in an ordinary way. This is paradise, radiant, blessed, the home of grace, and I can't take it with me when I return to my weighty, earthy, human existence. I know that now. The problems I left behind will still be knocking at my door. I understand that this spacious, love-filled realm of eternity belongs to gods and the world of time belongs to man and I am not a god.

E arly next morning begins with a knock on the hull.
'Hello. Je suis Kareen. I have come for the crew working. Je suis Francaise. Mon Anglais n'est pas bon.' She is pretty and thirty and wants to sail with Cornelius to Vanuatu.

'Have you done any sailing?' he asks.

'Bien sur, avec Jacques, son bateau s'appelle *Desperado*.'

Cornelius lights up. 'I know Jacques well. He's quite a womaniser. Where is he now?'

'Je ne sais pas. J'etais avec lui il y a deux ans.'

I reassure her that Cornelius is a fine man and a good sailor. I practice my rudimentary French: 'A demain nous allons a immigration.' Tomorrow Cornelius will sign her on as crew. What luck!

'Cornelius, we have to go now. It's late and I do want to go to Sigatoka. It's our last chance.'

Cornelius frowns then smiles, 'Sure.'

I turn to Kareen. 'We'll meet you at your hotel, ten o'clock tomorrow morning. Ca va? '

'Oui, parfait! A demain.' She leaves with a wave.

Well past noon, the bus to Nadi dumps us in a busy market swirling under clouds of grey diesel smoke. Locals crisscross in front of us, checking the produce piled high above the dusty gravel.

I shout in Cornelius's ear, 'I don't want to check my email. I'm going to the Hindu temple behind the town. We passed it on the way in. I'll meet you there.'

Cornelius frowns. 'Okay, I won't be long.'

T hirsty for inspiration, hungry for worldly confirmation of the spiritual, I set forth. My shaking head flicks off street hawkers like flies. I jaywalk intersections, speeding down the main road to a brightly-coloured, high-fenced Hindu place of worship. There I transition instantly into a state of expectant reverence. Brightly-painted wooden deities stand guard, protected from the rain in painted alcoves. I move around, looking for something more subtle. A central shrine? A complicated mix of oils and incense hangs in a doorway.

'Can I go in?' I ask the sleepy guard. He shakes his head and points away. I insist. Sleepy boredom is no match for me. I ask three times – he lets me pass.

Inside is fine and sweet smelling. Fraying silks wrap intricately-moulded copper and brass objects of devotion. Nothing is familiar. Will I be drawn instinctively to something? Maybe this many-headed brass figure sitting astride a grand peacock? I have no idea what it means. I want to feel devotional, but nothing moves inside me. My Tibetan Buddhist training was full of Taras, Chenrezigs and Manjusris. They sometimes had four arms, but only ever one head. The flowers and jewels and flowing robes were all symbols of precious qualities I was trying to instil in myself.

I lean against the glass cases and drift away. Years ago, on a two-month solo retreat, I used to walk in the bush every day, visualising myself as the deity Tara. Every day I chose a different symbol to work with: one day her silken flowing five-coloured gown, representing the five wisdoms, another day the white utpala flower she held to her heart, another day her brow, hands and feet enhanced with the seven eyes of wisdom. She was peaceful and smiling with the grace and charm of youth. Her back was supported by the full moon, and she was seated in the vajra position on a lotus flower resting on another full moon. These powerful images never left me for long. I held them as I walked, until they were my shaping, until I knew what they meant.

I don't know what anything means here. I'm on the outside, and from the outside this purpose and preoccupation seem childish, the symbols and rituals empty shells of a cultural idiosyncrasy. I walk back outside, quietly open to anything that might shift this cynical warp.

Near the outside wall of the shrine I stumble upon a hawk, its claws embedded in a pigeon. They stay still as can be, except for the eye of the hawk which follows me. I turn up some stairs and sit in the shade to watch. We stare at each other. Unexpectedly, Cornelius appears from the shadows and almost steps on the pair of birds. We look at each other and don't say anything. The hawk lets the pigeon go and flutters to a nearby roof where it continues to watch, hawk-eyed. The pigeon flutters from its pool of blood and feathers, out of sight. It doesn't try to escape the hawk – it's like they have a pact, a common destiny waiting to unfold. The hawk continues to watch us and it seems nothing will change until we move. I leave for my shoes and come across the pigeon, crouching underneath the hawk, bloodied brain oozing from its shattered head. Its death can be completed when we leave.

We put our shoes on, a little shaky. We had a good omen a month back – the fish leaping through the spreaders of Cornelius's boat. This is a bad omen.

A second bus drops us in Sigatoka. We start walking. I snuggle against his arm.

'What are the most important qualities in a relationship for you?' he asks as we pass some flowering bougainvillea. He answers because I don't. 'I think they are integrity and honesty.'

I slow down. 'What do you mean by integrity?'

'There's too much traffic, damn it. My shrink said integrity … '

I can't hear him for the traffic noise.

'Let's go across the bridge, away from the noise.' I pull his arm.

A footbridge with tracks for sugar cane trains spans the wide, slow-snaking Sigatoka River. We peer into the green water, reflecting afternoon light and distant hills and hanging branches. I weave romance into the dust and nailed-up windows of deserted houses. Indians and Fijians pass on their way home from work. Half way across the bridge I sit Cornelius down, legs through railway tracks, until we're like street urchins with nothing to do but watch the setting sun. He grumbles about dirt and grime on his clothes and hands. I disappear into the gloriously pink sky. Falling light silhouettes a large mosque on the hill and turns the river a pearly glow.

'Come on, let's go. I'm tired of this.' He gets up and brushes his trousers down.

We trudge the streets, turned shady now. A BBC newscast in a Chinese café presents Bush and Blair facing increasing criticism over their invasion of Iraq.

Cornelius gets up to pay the bill. 'Come on, I'm tired of this, too.'

We trudge back to the bus station through narrow, dark alleys. The last bus leaves in an hour. The light is hard and bare. Squalor breeds in the dark corners. A part of me leaps out with glee – I know who I am here, I feel at home. In the toilet, the smell of stale urine is asphyxiating. I could pass out before I open the door. I step with care, so I don't slip on the sticky, slippery floor. I lay Cornelius down on the bench seat to rest his leg, propping his head on my soft bag, then scamper off for cake, like a happy street urchin.

'This is my real home. This is me, inside out,' I boast, spitting crumbs, when I get back. He's not impressed. 'You asked if I was a bohemian, whether I lived outside the city walls. Well, actually I don't. I live in the gutters, I slip back and forth under the wall through sewer pipes. This bus stop is who I am.' He's not listening.

Our bus arrives and Cornelius stretches out on the back seat, head nestled in my lap. Passengers come on board and alight in the inky hours of blackness stretching out ahead of us. Cornelius moans for his leg. I swoon into the reflecting prism of our romance. The bus carries us safely home.

'Thank you for coming to Sigatoka with me. I know it was hard for you.' I kiss him good night.

Dad is anchored in Lautoka harbour. We are leaving in two days. A taxi drops Cornelius and me off at the wharf to meet his dinghy puttering into the rocks. He gets out slowly and climbs the stairs, head hanging low.

'Hi there,' I call.

His smile is rigid. 'Alice, you're not going to want to hear this, but I've changed my mind.' I stare at him, wondering what on earth he can mean. 'We're not going to Vanuatu after all. I want to stay in Fiji.'

I breathe deeply. I can't believe what I'm hearing. 'What! What do you mean?' I want to shake some sense into him.

'That's right. I don't want to go.'

I look at Cornelius. He doesn't speak.

'Dad, it's too late to change your mind.' I speak quietly. 'Kareen has cashed in her airplane ticket and signed on as crew with Cornelius at immigration. We have to go now.'

I know what he wants to say: "It's all your fault. I didn't want to go in the first place." I don't know if he actually said it. I have too many voices in my head screaming around.

'I want to stay here and meet a local woman so I can make some kind of a life. I won't be able to do that in Vanuatu.' His voice is flat and almost steady.

What can I do? Suddenly, I'm responsible for everything going wrong. It's all my fault. This is why I need my world to be perfect – I can't stand the weight when it crumbles, because it's not separated out from me properly, it's my own reflection – when it fails, I fail. My knees buckle and my hands go all clammy. Cornelius doesn't say anything.

The three of us stand together on the wharf, waiting for something to happen. I want to scream, "It's not fair! It's not my fault! I didn't want this to happen. I want us all to be happy."

'Cornelius, tell Dad that you have to sail to Vanuatu because of Kareen.'

'That's right, Roger.'

Dad is quiet, looking at his feet. He can't win, he's desperate. 'Okay, we'll go.'

'Come on, Dad, let's go out to *Dream-maker* and see what food we need.'

As planned I move onto *Dream-maker* to clean, buy food and prepare for the crossing. We work together in slow motion, the hint of a truce, doing what needs to be done, sharing meals, fitting back together.

Cornelius and I go out to dinner on our last night together in Fiji, my forty-eighth birthday. Twinkling coloured lights strung along open thatched roofs recreate an atmosphere of romantic fantasy. The bare bulbs create shadows. The mix is confusing. The wine makes me careless.

Cornelius brushes past, shouting in a hoarse whisper, 'You're too much of a risk to be trusted. You're just like my mother!' and slips out the back with the waitress. I burst into a sweat, wet stone. Candles flicker above the cake placed in front of me. 'Happy birthday to you … ' they sing.

I don't sleep for the faces swirling in my mind – ugly demented faces with long stringy arms and claws, reaching up out of sewer grates.

We taxi around to Lautoka wharf the next morning. Dad is waiting.

'I'll be leaving in three days. I might even catch you up,' Cornelius brags.

'I do hope so.' My arms lock around him, not wanting to let go. 'I'll radio you at nine every morning and evening – channel 7260.'

I stare into his eyes, happy and sad.

He holds my face, hands soft on my cheeks, and kisses me. My heart flutters – he still loves me, we'll be okay. I follow my bags down into the dinghy, Dad pulls the starting cord, the motor bursts into life and we're off. Cornelius climbs into the waiting taxi and doesn't look back.

THE
ANCHORS IN AN OPEN SEA
TRILOGY
Sailing into the full catastrophe of living

Have you ever wondered what it is like to be driven for most of your life by an overwhelming desire for spiritual experience?

Explore with Alice through thirty tumultuous years, cycling, tramping, sailing, making love, attending spiritual retreats, raising a family and eventually teaching. Taste life through mystical eyes, experience being raised to heaven and the torment of being plunged to earth when the heart fails.

Endlessly curious about life and the human journey, Alice throws herself with abandon into the natural world, rough and raw, creating heroic confusion as she plunges deeply into the mystery of mind. What she discovers at the end is not what she expected.

This is your chance to travel with her and come to understand why her desire for spiritual experience was so overwhelming, and why she found it so hard to make peace with ordinary living.

The autobiographical honesty and poetical language make this story compelling. Hang on as you sail off with Alice into the ocean with its stunning sunsets and tumultuous waves.

http://dyanawells.com

http://fieryscribes.com

BOOK TWO

BUDDHA AND A BOAT

Digging into the mystery when life gets sticky

Alice, Roger and Cornelius set sail from Fiji for Vanuatu and New Caledonia and the adventure and excitement continue. They share watches through the day and night, cope with seasickness, struggle with headwinds, and Cornelius is almost immobilised with an unexplained pain in his leg.

When she goes cycling solo around Vanuatu, Alice explores teachings from earlier retreats and she reflects on her early life as she hitches alone around New Caledonia. She is swept into the lives of a local Kanak family. She starts to see why she is the way she is. When some of the family visit from New Zealand, the pressure builds to explosive and she falls apart.

We also see Alice as an older woman – softer and wiser. She is with her children, who are now almost the age she was when she went sailing. She has a deeper perspective, and we see that she has succeeded in bringing her two worlds together. We don't know how she did it, or exactly what that means, but we do see that she is different, and that she has something to share.

http://dyanawells.com

http://fieryscribes.com

BOOK THREE
MY TRUE NAMES
Standing in the presence of our daemons

Alice and Cornelius begin the adventure of a lifetime, sailing from Fiji through Vanuatu and the Solomon archipelago on to the islands of Papua New Guinea. The pristine waters abound with tropical fish and coral, the volcanic islands are alive with gardens and lush jungle.

Alice wants to keep sailing forever, in spite of serious relationship difficulties. She repeats her mantra – stay present and be interested. Of course she fails, most often she fails, and yet she knows that until she comes close to what frightens her the most, until she befriends her most difficult moments, whatever she found that was valuable in her mystical adventures will be lost. She has everything to gain and everything to lose.

The older, wiser Alice is now teaching, incorporating neurophysiological models of consciousness. Her daughter Charlotte, thoroughly dispirited about what humans do to themselves and others, comes to study with her. Alice introduces her to the Foundation Teaching of Buddhism and Tantric Creative Visualisation, so that Charlotte too may accept this human life and work for the benefit of all beings.

http://dyanawells.com

http://fieryscribes.com

DYANA WELLS

Dyana's life has always been shaped around a few central questions: Who am I? What is this thing called life? What am I meant to be doing with my life? These questions seem to be without final answers but capable of revealing ever deepening insights into the mystery of living. They have taken her on many remarkable adventures. Maybe the best words to describe Dyana would be mystical scientist.

These books describe her journey into the confusion and the extraordinary love and fulfilment of the spiritual quest. She investigates in a raw way the difficulties and distortions that mystical experience can create.

Dyana runs regular workshops integrating Mind-Body, Meditation and Buddhist philosophy and currently teaches Yoga Philosophy and Anatomy & Physiology to Contemporary Yoga Teacher trainees in Auckland, New Zealand.

She has three children and four grandchildren and lives at Orere Point, a small seaside village outside Auckland.

http://dyanawells.com

http://fieryscribes.com